Contents

A

B

C

D

E

F

G

H

O

P

R

S

X

A

NORMAL VALUES

Average value: 25–39 seconds

Purpose of the Test

This test measures the time needed for a clot to form. The aPTT is used to help identify deficiencies of coagulation. It is also used to monitor the effect of heparin therapy that is administered by intermittent injection and to adjust the dosage of the drug based on the test results. The therapeutic range for heparinization is 1 1/2 to 2 times the control or normal value.

Procedure

A blue-topped tube with sodium citrate is used to obtain 4.5 ml of venous blood. As an alternative, a heelstick, earlobe, or finger puncture may be used to collect capillary blood in siliconized sodium citrate micropipettes.

✓ QUALITY CONTROL
The tube must be filled with blood. If filling is incomplete, the increased concentration of sodium citrate will cause a false elevation of the test result.

To mix the sodium citrate with the blood, the specimen tube is tilted gently from side to side, 5 to 10 times.

When multiple specimens are drawn, the aPTT test specimen is obtained last, using a double tube technique. A 1 to 2 ml blood sample is obtained and discarded; the blue-topped tube is then used to collect the test sample.

To prevent hemolysis and a false decrease in the test result, venipuncture technique must be smooth, with a blood flow that fills the vacuum tube readily.

Findings

Increase	*Decrease*
Excess administration of heparin	Hypercoagulable states (with recurring arterial or venous thrombus formation)
Abnormality of the coagulation system	
Disseminated intravascular coagulation (DIC)	
Liver failure with vitamin K deficiency	

Interfering Factors

Hemolysis
Inadequate blood sample
Prolonged delay before analysis is performed

Nursing Implementation

- *Pretest*

When heparin is given in intermittent doses, ensure that the specimen is drawn 1 hour before the next dose. When heparin is given in a continuous infusion, special timing of the test is unnecessary.

- *During the Test*

Ensure that the heparin lock or a heparinized catheter is not used to obtain the blood specimen.

- *Posttest*

Arrange for prompt transport of the specimen to the laboratory.

✓ QUALITY CONTROL
Specimens received more than 2 hours after collection will be rejected because the plasma must be separated from the cells and refrigerated as soon as possible.

When the patient receives heparin anticoagulation therapy, monitor each aPTT result for a value in the therapeutic range. The possible panic value is 70 second or above. If an aPTT result is very elevated, notify the physician immediately. Protamine sulfate, IM, is the antidote to heparin.

ADRENOCORTICOTROPIC HORMONE • PLASMA

Synonym: ACTH

NORMAL VALUES

In a.m.: 25–100 pg/ml *or* SI 25–100 ng/L
In p.m.: 0–50 pg/ml *or* SI 0–50 ng/L

Purpose of the Test

Adrenocorticotropic hormone (ACTH) is produced and secreted by the anterior pituitary gland. Its secretion is under the control of the hypothalamus and the central nervous system by neurotransmitters and corticotropin-releasing hormone (CRH). ACTH, in turn, regulates the secretion of the glucocorticoids and androgens from the adrenal cortex. An increase or decrease in the production of ACTH will cause an increase or decrease in the glucocorticoid levels. A deficiency of ACTH will cause secondary adrenal insufficiency. An increase in ACTH will cause Cushing's disease (Cushing's syndrome is a primary adrenal disorder).

A plasma ACTH determination is obtained to diagnose Cushing's disease and differentiate primary and secondary adrenal insufficiency.

Procedure

Venipuncture is required to obtain 1 ml of venous blood in a heparinized green-topped tube. The plasma ACTH is measured by RIA.

Findings

Increase

Primary adrenal insufficiency
Cushing's disease
Congenital adrenal hyperplasia
Ectopic ACTH syndrome

Decrease

Primary adrenal hypersecretion
Cushing's syndrome

Tumors of the adrenal gland may suppress the ACTH level if they produce glucocorticoids; however, not all adrenal tumors do.

Interfering Factors

Noncompliance with medication, diet, or activity restrictions
Administration of radioactive scans within 7 days
Pregnancy
Ingestion of alcohol
Amphetamines
Calcium gluconate
Corticosteroids
Estrogen
Lithium
Spironolactone

Nursing Implementation

• Pretest

Explain to the patient about the need to obtain two specimens of blood, one in the early morning (6 to 8 a.m.) and one in the evening (6 to 11 p.m.). The early morning specimen reflects the peak secretion time and the evening specimen the low secretion period for ACTH.

Instruct the patient to ingest nothing by mouth for 12 hours before the test. Some physicians recommend a low-carbohydrate diet for 2 days before the test.

Obtain a medication history and question prescriber if any interfering drugs should be withheld.

Inquire and note on requisition slip if the patient is pregnant, as this may affect test results.

• During the Test

After blood is obtained by venipuncture, place the specimen on ice and immediately send to the laboratory.

Notify laboratory personnel that the specimen is being transported, as it should be frozen until an RIA can be performed.

• Posttest

The patient resumes a normal diet, activity, and medication regimen.

ALANINE AMINOTRANSFERASE (ALT) • SERUM

N O R M A L   V A L U E S

Adult: 10–35 IU/L at 37° C
Newborn–1 year: 13–45 IU/L at 37° C

Purpose of the Test

The alanine aminotransferase test detects the rise of transaminase enzymes that results from injury or necrosis of the liver. Very severe elevations indicate acute hepatitis. Moderate elevations indicate other causes of liver disease.

Procedure

Venipuncture is performed to obtain 5 to 10 ml of blood in a red-topped tube.

✓ QUALITY CONTROL
To prevent hemolysis of erythrocytes, venipuncture technique must be smooth, with a blood flow that fills the vacutainer tube readily.

Findings

Increase

Acute hepatitis
Cirrhosis
Obstructive jaundice
Liver tumor

Interfering Factors

Hemolysis

Nursing Implementation

• *Pretest*

Many medications cause an elevated test result. If they cannot be discontinued for 12 hours, list the patient's medications on the requisition slip.

ALKALINE PHOSPHATASE (ALP) • SERUM

NORMAL VALUES

Adult: 4.5–13 King-Armstrong units/dL *or* SI 32–92 UL
       1.4–4.4 Bodansky units
Infant: 10–30 King-Armstrong units/dL *or* SI 71–213 UL

Purpose of the Test

Serum alkaline phosphatase provides a nonspecific indicator of liver disease, bone disease, or hyperparathyroidism. It is part of the battery of tests that evaluates liver function. It also serves as a nonspecific tumor marker, indicating rapid cell growth or accelerated function due to malignancy of the liver or bone.

Procedure

A red-topped sterile tube is used to collect 5 to 10 ml of venous blood.

✓ QUALITY CONTROL
In the laboratory, the serum must be kept refrigerated until analyzed. Heat, warmth, or prolonged storage of the specimen will falsely elevate the results.

Findings

Increase

Cancer (liver, bone, pancreas, or bone marrow)
Paget's disease
Biliary obstruction
Cirrhosis
Infiltrating liver disease (infection, sarcoidosis)
Rickets
Hyperparathyroidism
Hyperthyroidism
Acromegaly

Decrease

Malnutrition (protein and/or magnesium deficiency)
Hypophosphatemia
Hypothyroidism

Interfering Factors

Pregnancy
Healing bone fracture
Fatty food intake 2 to 4 hours before the test

Nursing Implementation

• *Pretest*

Instruct the patient to discontinue food intake for 12 hours before the test, according to laboratory policy. Foods in general and fatty foods in particular can elevate the test results in some people.

ALPHA₁ FETOPROTEIN (AFP)   • SERUM

NORMAL VALUES

Adult: 2–16 ng/ml *or* SI 2–16 µg/L
Normal pregnancy (third trimester): 550 ng/ml *or* SI: 550 µg/L

Purpose of the Test

In nonpregnant adults, this test is used as a tumor marker for particular types of malignancy and to monitor the tumor's response to antineoplastic medication.

In the 16th to 18th weeks of pregnancy, this test is used to screen for particular types of congenital defects in the fetus. Elevated results require additional testing, such as ultrasound and amniotic fluid analysis.

Procedure

A red-topped sterile tube is used to collect 5 to 10 ml of venous blood.

✓ QUALITY CONTROL
The specimen is kept refrigerated until the analysis is performed.

Findings

Increase

Nonpregnancy
Gonadal germinal tumor
Primary cancer of the liver
Cancer of the pancreas, gall
   bladder, bile duct, or
   stomach

Pregnancy
Spina bifida
Myelomeningocele
Anencephaly
Fetal death

Interfering Factors

Recent radioisotope scan

Nursing Implementation

• *Pretest*

On the requisition slip of the pregnant patient, include the following data: gestational age, maternal weight, race, and diabetic status.

> ✓ QUALITY CONTROL
> These are variables that affect the interpretation of normal values.

• *Posttest*

If the patient is informed of the abnormal result and the possible significance, provide appropriate support to help the patient cope with anxiety and fear. Additional testing is needed to investigate the cause of the elevated value.

AMMONIA (NH) • SERUM

N O R M A L   V A L U E S

Adult: 15–45 µg/L *or* SI 11–22 µmol/L
Child: 29–70 µg/dl *or* SI 21–50 µmol/L
Neonate: 90–150 µg/dl *or* SI 64–107 µmol/L

Purpose of the Test

The ammonia level is used to evaluate or monitor severe liver failure, hepatoencephalopathy, and the effects of impaired portal vein circulation.

Procedure

A gray, lavender, or green-topped sterile tube is used to collect 3 to 5 ml of venous blood.

✓ QUALITY CONTROL
The vacuum tube must be fully filled and then kept sealed to prevent a false positive result. Once the blood is drawn, the vial must be placed on ice and rotated immediately to chill the specimen.

Findings

Increase

Liver failure
Cirrhosis
Hepatoencephalopathy
Portal hypertension
Aminoaciduria
Reye's Syndrome

Interfering Factors

Tobacco smoke
High protein intake
Gastrointestinal hemorrhage
Hyperalimentation
Ureterosigmoidostomy

Nursing Implementation

• *Pretest*

Instruct the patient to fast from food for 8 hours prior to the test because protein intake would raise the ammonia level. Water intake is permitted.

Instruct the patient not to smoke before the test, since the smoke itself will alter the results.

• *Posttest*

Insure that the vial of blood is kept on ice and is sent to the laboratory immediately.

✓ QUALITY CONTROL
To avoid false positive results, the serum must be analyzed or frozen within 20 minutes.

AMNIOCENTESIS • AMNIOTIC FLUID

N O R M A L   V A L U E S

AMNIOTIC FLUID ANALYSIS
Chromosomal analysis: Normal characteristics
Alpha$_1$-fetoprotein: 0.5–3 MoM
Bilirubin: 0.01–0.03 mg/dl *or* SI 0.02–0.06 µmol/L
Lecithin/sphingomyelin ratio: >2
Phosphatidylglycerol: Present
Meconium: Negative

Purpose of the Test

Early analysis detects genetic or chromosomal abnormalities in the fetus. In the management of a problem pregnancy, it is used to assess fetal maturity or fetal distress.

Procedure

Amniocentesis is performed to obtain the sample of amniotic fluid. Several syringes and a long needle are used to aspirate 10 to 20 ml of amniotic fluid from the uterus. The fluid is placed in sterile brown plastic containers.

✓ QUALITY CONTROL
Glass containers cannot be used because cells adhere to the surface of the glass. An amber-colored container is used to protect the solution and bilirubin from the sunlight.

Findings

Abnormal

Chromosomal defect
Down syndrome
Cystic fibrosis
Sickle cell anemia

Increase

Alpha₁-fetoprotein
Anencephaly
Spina bifida
Myelocele
Hydrocephaly
Congenital nephrosis
Esophageal atresia
Bilirubin
Rh incompatibility
L/S ratio
Maternal diabetes
Meconium
Fetal distress

Decrease

Bilirubin
Fetal immaturity
L/S ratio
Fetal pulmonary immaturity
Phosphatidylglycerol
Fetal pulmonary immaturity

Interfering Factors

Exposure of specimen to sunlight
Contamination of specimen (blood, meconium)
Recent radioactive isotope scan
Position of the placenta
Delay in delivery of specimen to laboratory

Nursing Implementation

- *Pretest*

After the patient receives a complete explanation of the amniocentesis procedure from the physician, obtain her written consent.

Provide instructions regarding pretest preparation. For a pregnancy that is less than 20 weeks of gestation, the woman drinks extra fluids 1 hour before the test and does not urinate until the test is completed. For a pregnancy that is greater than 20 weeks of gestation, there are no requirements for fluid intake. Instruct the woman to void before the procedure begins.

Obtain and record the blood pressure, temperature, pulse, respirations, and fetal heart rate.

Provide emotional support because anxiety about the procedure and the baby are common.

- *During the Test*

Position the patient on the table, with her hands behind her head. Wash the abdomen with providone-iodine solution and drape the sterile field.

Comfort the patient during the injection of the local anesthetic. Some stinging may be felt.

After the fluid sample is withdrawn, assist with its placement in the specimen containers.

Once the needle is withdrawn, place a small adhesive bandage over the site of the needle puncture.

- *Posttest*

Monitor and record the blood pressure, pulse, respirations, and fetal heart rate every 15 minutes for 30 to 60 minutes.

Ensure that the specimen is correctly labeled. The requisition slip should state the source of the fluid and the period of gestation of the pregnancy.

If the patient feels faintness, nausea, or cramps, place her on her right side to relieve the uterine pressure.

At the time of discharge, instruct the patient to rest at home until the cramping subsides. Light activity can then resume. Heavy lifting or strenuous activity is avoided for several days.

Provide the patient with written instructions to notify the physician immediately about any symptoms of itching, fever, leakage of fluid, severe abdominal pain, or unusual (increased or decreased) fetal activity.

✪ **COMPLICATION ALERT** ✪ In addition to assessing for signs of infection (fever or purulence) and bleeding (hematoma) at the puncture site, the nurse should remain alert for potential changes in the fetus (lethargy or hyperactivity) and uterus (leakage of fluid from the vagina or severe persistant uterine contractions).

AMYLASE • SERUM, URINE

NORMAL VALUES

SERUM
Adult: 24–151 U/L *or* SI 0.41–2.57 µKat/L
Neonate: 5–65 U/L *or* 0.09–1.11 µKat/L

URINE
Adult: 4–30 IU/2 hours (2-hour test)
Up to 3000 units/24 hours (24-hour test)

Purpose of the Test

Serum amylase is used to investigate the cause of severe abdominal or epigastric pain, particularly when acute pancreatic disorder is suspected. It may also be used to evaluate pancreatic dysfunction in cases of severe cystic fibrosis.

Urine amylase helps to diagnose acute pancreatitis when the serum levels are borderline or normal.

Procedure

Serum

A red-topped sterile tube is used to collect 5 to 10 ml of venous blood.

Urine

Urine is collected in a clean container for the prescribed time period of 2, 6, 8, or 24 hours.

✓ QUALITY CONTROL
Personnel should not talk, sneeze, or cough near either type of open specimen. Their saliva will add to the amylase content of the specimen.

Findings

Increase	*Decrease*
Acute pancreatitis	Chronic pancreatitis
Pancreatic disorder (trauma, abscess, cancer)	Cystic fibrosis
Obstruction of the pancreatic duct	Pancreatic cancer

Interfering Factors

Serum	*Urine*
Ingestion of alcohol	Ingestion of alcohol
Narcotic medications	Contamination of the specimen by menstrual flow or salivary amylase
	Omission of any voided specimen
	Failure to cool the specimen

Nursing Implementation

- *Pretest*

Serum

Drugs (morphine, Demerol, codeine) that affect amylase levels may be omitted or postponed.

Urine

Just before the start of the test, instruct the patient to void and discard the specimen. This urine has been in the bladder for an unknown time period. Then start the timing of the test.

Serum and Urine

Inform the patient to avoid alcohol ingestion for 24 hours before the test. Alcohol stimulates the secretion of salivary amylase.

- *During the Test*

Urine

All specimens are collected and added to the clean urine container, including the final voided urine of the time period.

Refrigerate the container of urine or place the container in a basin of ice. Amylase is very unstable in acidic urine.

On the specimen label and requisition slip, write the date and time of the start and the finish of the test.

ANGIOGRAPHY, BRAIN, HEAD, AND NECK
• RADIOGRAPHY

Synonym: Cerebral angiography

N O R M A L   V A L U E S
No abnormalities of the tissue or vasculature are visualized.

Purpose of the Test

Angiography of the brain, head, and neck provides clear imaging of intracranial and extracranial vascular abnormalities and their locations. Although the less invasive procedure of computed tomography (CT) has surpassed angiography for the imaging of tumors and trauma to the brain, angiography remains a mainstay in the investigation of the cerebral vasculature. There are several different types of cerebral angiography that can be performed.

In addition to the visualization of the vasculature of the head, neck, and brain, cerebral angiography demonstrates the location and characteristic vascular patterns of different types of brain tumors. It locates and defines the source of a subarachnoid hemorrhage and also identifies vascular malformation. Thrombosis, embolic occlusion, or atheromatous stenosis can be seen when it occurs in a major extracranial or intracranial artery. Subdural hematoma is also visualized because there is no contrast material circulating in the space between the skull and the displaced brain tissue.

Procedure

Iodinated radiopaque contrast material is injected arterially or intravenously. Rapid serial x-ray films are taken to image the bolus of contrast medium as it moves through the circulation of the neck and extracranial and intracranial blood vessels.

Findings

Brain tumor
Fistula
Arteriovenous malformation
Obstruction of the cerebrospinal fluid
Arteriosclerosis
Atherosclerotic plaque
Cerebral aneurysm

Cerebral edema
Subarachnoid hemorrhage
Stenosis
Vascular occlusion

Interfering Factors

Movement of the head during imaging
Metal objects in the x-ray field
Allergy to iodine

Nursing Implementation

- *Pretest*

Ask the patient about history of previous allergy to iodine, including an allergic reaction to seafood, shellfish, or iodine
during previous x-ray studies using contrast medium.

Obtain written consent from the patient or the person who
has legal responsibility for the patient's health care decisions.

Instruct the patient regarding the food and fluid restrictions
before the test. Because there are some variations among institutions, verify the protocol that is to be used by the particular radiology department.

Instruct the patient to discontinue food intake for 6 to 8 hours
before the test. The contrast medium can cause nausea. If
there is food in the stomach, the vomiting would result in
head movement during the imaging process and blurring of
the photographic results.

Most institutions permit the intake of clear fluids during the
fasting period. Some limit the amount and others encourage
extra intake of fluids to promote hydration and renal excretion of the contrast medium. For the patient who has fluid
restrictions, intravenous fluids are started early in the test period so that renal function is optimal.

When this test is to be performed on an outpatient or ambulatory basis, instruct the patient to have a responsible person
available for transportation home after the test. The sedative
effects of the medications will remain for several hours after
the test is completed.

Assist the patient in removing all clothing and putting on a hospital gown. All metal objects and jewelry are removed from head, hair, neck, and upper torso.

Inform the patient that he or she may feel a temporary flushing or burning sensation, a salty taste, headache, or nausea as the contrast medium is injected.

Take the baseline vital signs and assess movement of extremities. Record the results.

Administer the prescribed pretest sedative and analgesic medications. The purposes of the medications are to decrease central nervous system activity, anxiety, tension, physical activity, and potential agitation. Some of the medications also reduce nausea and the potential for vomiting. The particular combination of drugs varies with the institutional protocol or choice of the physician.

• *During the Test*

Establish an intravenous line for fluid replacement and the electrocardiographic leads for monitoring the heart rate and rhythm. Take vital signs at appropriate intervals.

Instruct the patient to keep the head and neck absolutely still during the injection of contrast material and the imaging sequence.

Restraints may be used to prevent movement.

• *Posttest*

Once the catheter is removed from the artery, use sterile gauze to apply digital pressure to the puncture site for 10 minutes. This should prevent bleeding or hematoma formation. If swelling or redness occurs, apply ice to the area.

Continue to monitor vital signs at frequent intervals until they are stable.

Assess the patient's mental status, observing for clarity of thinking, alertness, and intact neurologic function.

Prior to discharge, instruct the patient to remain on bedrest for the remainder of the day. By the next day, most physical activities may be resumed, but vigorous exercise should be avoided for an additional day or two.

Observe for neurologic deficit, stroke, excessive bleeding, and reaction to contrast dye.

✪ COMPLICATION ALERT ✪ The nurse must maintain close observation of the patient for a minimum of 2 hours for this is when most of the complications occur.

ANGIOSCOPY • ENDOSCOPY

Synonym: Vascular endoscopy

NORMAL VALUES

The lumen of the artery or bypass graft is free from obstruction. The suture line is intact, and the graft is patent.

Purpose of the Test

Angioscopy is used to visualize the lumen and endothelial surfaces of the affected artery or vein directly so that the cause of the obstruction or impaired blood flow can be identified.

Angioscopy is usually performed as an adjunctive procedure during vascular surgery. It provides direct visualization and monitors the vascular surgical interventions; such as, bypass grafting, endarterectomy, thrombectomy, embolectomy, angioplasty, or closed repair of a blood vessel. On completion of a saphenous vein bypass graft, the angioscope is passed through the graft to inspect the lumen and distal anastomosis. After thrombectomy or atherectomy, the angioscope is used to inspect the lumen for residual fragments of plaque or clots. Residual particles are removed or the graft is revised, as necessary.

The use of angioscopy has expanded as a diagnostic procedure, because angioscopes can be inserted percutaneously. Percutaneous angioscopy of pulmonary, peripheral, and coronary arteries is part of an experimental protocol in some medical centers.

Procedure

Angioscopes are small, flexible endoscopes of different diameters designed to fit into narrow vessels. The angioscope contains fiberoptics and a light source for visualization of the obstruction. A videocamera is connected to the viewing eyepiece, and the images of the lumen are projected onto a videomonitor. Within the angioscopy, there is an irrigation-instrumentation channel to remove blood from the lens, and small instruments can incise, suture, or remove small sources of obstruction.

The angioscope is inserted through a small surgical opening in the artery or vein and is passed into the lumen in an antegrade or retrograde direction. This may be performed through the skin (percutaneous approach) or through an open surgical incision.

Findings

Severe peripheral vascular disease
Residual valve leaflets in the venous bypass graft
Bypass graft torsion (twisting) or stenosis
Arterial thrombus or embolus
Platelet thrombus
Incompetent venous valve leaflets

Interfering Factors

None

Nursing Implementation

• *Pretest*

Provide preoperative instructions and obtain a written consent from the patient or person legally responsible for health care decisions.

Instruct the patient to ingest nothing by mouth for 8 hours before the test or surgery.

Collect baseline data and record the results in the patient's chart. These data include determinations of blood pressure, pulse, respirations, and appropriate peripheral pulses (those distal to the area of arterial surgery and angioscopy).

Administer the prescribed sedative analgesic for relaxation.

• *During the Test*

Connect and test all equipment prior to the start of the procedure. The videocamera is focused correctly.

Maintain and replace the supply of irrigation fluid, preventing air bubbles from entering the system or the patient's circulation.

Record the total volume of irrigation fluid used. The irrigation fluid volume should be included in the patient's intake.

✓ QUALITY CONTROL
The angioscope is cleaned, wrapped, and gas-sterilized after each use to prevent transmission of infection and the onset of sepsis.

• *Posttest*

Observe the surgical or arteriotomy incision for signs of localized swelling, hematoma formation, or bleeding. When a percutaneous approach is used, the incision may be small.

Observe and assess the distal extremity for color, temperature, and the presence of pulses.

ANGIOTENSIN-CONVERTING ENZYME   • SERUM

Synonyms: ACE, serum angiotensin-converting enzyme, SACE

N O R M A L   V A L U E S

ADULT*
Male: 12–36 IU/L *or* SI same
Female: 10–30 IU/L *or* SI same

*Norms for individuals younger than 20 years of age are slightly higher.

Purpose of the Test

ACE levels are determined to evaluate hypertension and to diagnose and treat sarcoidosis.

Procedure

A venipuncture is performed to collect 5 ml of blood in a red-topped tube.

Findings

Increase

Cirrhosis
Gaucher's disease (familial
    disorder of fat metabolism)
Hansen's disease
Histoplasmosis
Hodgkin's disease
Hyperthyroidism
Myeloma
Pulmonary fibrosis
Sarcoidosis
Scleroderma

Decrease

Adult respiratory distress syn-
    drome
Diabetes mellitus
Hypothyroidism
Tuberculosis

Interfering Factors

Steroids

Nursing Implementation

The nursing actions are similar to those for other venipuncture
procedures.

ANION GAP • SERUM

Synonyms: None

N O R M A L   V A L U E S
10–15 mEq/L *or* SI 10–15 µmol/L

Purpose of the Test

The anion gap is the sum of unmeasured anions in the serum:
phosphates, sulfates, ketones, proteins, and organic acids. It is
used to distinguish among causes of metabolic acidosis. Patients
with diabetic ketoacidosis usually have a large anion gap, whereas
those with metabolic acidosis due to intestinal fluid loss have a
nearly normal anion gap. The anion gap is calculated to determine the cause of metabolic acidosis.

Procedure

The anion gap is determined by subtracting the sum of measured anions (bicarbonate [HCO_3] and chloride [Cl]) from the measured cations (sodium [Na] and potassium [K]).

Findings

Increase

Hypernatremia
Hyperosmolar coma
Hypocalcemia
Hypomagnesemia
Ketoacidosis
Lactic acidosis
Starvation

Decrease

Hypercalcemia
Hypermagnesemia
Hypoalbuminemia
Hyponatremia
Multiple myeloma

Interfering Factors

Dehydration
Ingestion of licorice
Excessive ingestion of antacids
Ethylene glycol
Methanol
Paraldehyde
Salicylates
Medications (partial listing: adrenocorticotropic hormone, antihypertensive agents, bicarbonates, chlorpropamide, diuretics, lithium, steroids, vasopressin)

Nursing Implementation

After the results of blood electrolyte determinations are obtained, calculate the anion gap during the test with the following formula:

$$(Na + K) - (HCO_3 + Cl) = \text{anion gap}$$

ANTIGLOBULIN, DIRECT, INDIRECT (COOMBS, DIRECT, INDIRECT) • BLOOD

NORMAL VALUES

Negative

Purpose of the Test

The antiglobulin tests detect antibodies on the erythrocytes and in the serum. They are used in type and crossmatch testing and in evaluation of a blood transfusion reaction caused by incompatibility. They are used in the diagnosis and treatment of maternal–fetal blood incompatibility and also help to diagnose hemolytic anemia.

Procedure

Direct Antiglobulin

One red-topped and one lavender-topped tube are used to collect 7 ml of venous blood in each tube. In the newborn, venous cord blood may be collected.

Indirect Antiglobulin

A red-topped tube is used to collect 7 ml of venous blood.

> ✓ QUALITY CONTROL
> To prevent hemolysis or clumping of erythrocytes, the tourniquet must not be applied tightly or for a prolonged time. Venipuncture technique must be smooth, with a blood flow that fills the tube readily.

Findings

Increase

Direct antiglobulin test
Autoimmune hemolytic anemia
Hemolytic transfusion reaction
Hemolytic disease of the newborn
Sensitivity to particular medications (methyldopa [Aldomet], levodopa [Dopar], and others)
Indirect antiglobulin test
Maternal–fetal blood incompatibility
Autoimmune hemolytic anemia
Sensitivity to particular medications (methyldopa [Aldomet], levodopa [Dopar], and others)

Interfering Factors

Hemolysis
Inadequate identification of the specimen

Nursing Implementation

• *Pretest*

On the requisition form, include any recent history of blood transfusion or plasma expanders and a list of medications taken.

• *Posttest*

Ensure that the specimen and requisition slip include the patient's name, identification number, and the source of the blood (venous, cord).

Arrange for prompt transport of the specimen to the laboratory.

ANTINUCLEAR ANTIBODY • SERUM

Synonyms: ANA, fluorescent antinuclear antibody, FANA, ANF

NORMAL VALUES

Negative at a 1:20 dilution

Purpose of the Test

The ANA test is used as a screen to detect autoimmune disease or systemic lupus erythematosus, or both. With the ANA test, the analysis consists of microscopic examination of the serum for the presence of immunofluorescent-stained antigen-antibody complexes. Additionally, the amount of antibody is measured by the presence of a high serum titer. Positive ANA results identify the presence of the antitissue antibodies of autoimmune disease, but it cannot identify the specific disease. As a screening tool, however, ANA is particularly relevant in the detection of systemic lupus erythematosus because of a higher accuracy rate in detection of this particular antibody. It is also used to monitor the effectiveness of medication in the treatment of systemic lupus erythematosus.

Procedure

A red-topped tube is used to collect 7 to 10 ml of venous blood.

✓ QUALITY CONTROL
Venipuncture technique must be smooth, with a blood flow that fills the vacuum tube rapidly. If the blood has excessive turbulence because of flawed venipuncture technique, the hemolysis of the erythrocytes will alter test results.

Findings

Increase

Systemic autoimmune diseases

Systemic lupus erythematosus
Rheumatoid arthritis
Ankylosing spondylitis
Necrotizing angiitis
Polymyositis
Dermatomyositis
Progressive systemic sclerosis
Mixed connective tissue disease
Sjögren's syndrome

Autoimmune diseases of blood and target organs

Hashimoto's thyroiditis
Myxedema
Thyrotoxicosis
Hepatic or biliary cirrhosis
Leukemia
Chronic renal failure
Multiple sclerosis
Pernicious anemia
Regional ileitis
Ulcerative colitis
Gluten-sensitive enteropathy
Pemphigus vulgaris

Interfering Factors

Hemolysis of the blood specimen

Nursing Implementation

• *Pretest*

List any medications taken by the patient.

• *Posttest*

Arrange for prompt transport of the specimen to the laboratory. The cells must be extracted from the serum promptly to prevent contamination of the specimen because of hemolysis.

ARTERIAL BLOOD GASES • ARTERIAL BLOOD

Synonym: ABGs

NORMAL VALUES

pH: 7.35–7.45 *or* SI 7.35–7.45
Pco$_2$: 35–45 mm Hg *or* SI 4.7–5.3 kPa
HCO3: 21–28 mEq/L *or* SI 21–28 μmol/L
Po$_2$
Adult: 80–100 mm Hg *or* SI 10.6–13.3 kPa
Newborn: 60–70 mm Hg *or* SI 8.0–10.33 kPa
Sao$_2$
Adult: >95% *or* SI fraction saturated >0.95
Newborn: 40–90% *or* SI fraction saturated 0.40–0.90
Base excess: ± 2 mEq/L *or* SI ± 2 μmol/L

Purpose of the Test

ABG determinations are obtained for a variety of reasons, including the diagnosis of chronic and restrictive pulmonary disease, adult respiratory failure, acid-base disturbances, pulmonary emboli, sleep disorders, central nervous system dysfunctions, and cardiovascular disorders such as congestive heart failure, shunts, and intracardiac atrial or ventricular shunts, or both.

Arterial blood gases are used in the management of patients on mechanical ventilators and during the weaning process from the ventilators.

Procedure

An arterial blood sample of 5 ml is obtained via an arterial puncture or arterial line. The radial or femoral artery is usually used in adults, whereas the temporal artery is used in infants.

Findings

Hypoxia

Respiratory acidosis (low pH, high pCO$_2$): Respiratory center dysfunction (opiates, anesthetics, sedatives, oxygen-induced hypoventilation, central nervous system lesions), disorders of the respiratory muscles or chest wall (myasthenia gravis, amyotrophic lateral sclerosis, kyphoscoliosis, Pickwickian syndrome, splinting due to pain), disorders of gas exchange (chronic lung disease, acute pulmonary edema, asphyxia), hypoventilation while on a mechanical ventilator

Respiratory alkalosis (high pH, low pCO_2): Hyperventilation (atelectasis, severe anemia, pulmonary emboli, anxiety), central nervous system disorders (brain stem dysfunction, subarachnoid hemorrhage), salicylate poisoning, hypermetabolic states (fever, thyrotoxicosis, sepsis), hyperventilation while on mechanical ventilation

Metabolic acidosis (low pH, low HCO_3): Diabetic ketoacidosis, lactic acidosis, excessive ingestion of acid (salicylates, ethylene, methanol, paraldehyde), loss of bicarbonate (diarrhea, fistulas), renal failure

Metabolic alkalosis (high pH, high HCO_3): Loss of body acid (vomiting, excessive gastric suctioning), excessive diuresis, hypokalemia, excessive ingestion of licorice, nonparathyroid hypercalcemia, HCO_3 overload (excessive ingestion of bicarbonate, massive blood transfusions)

Interfering Factors

Noncompliance with proper collection procedure, including air bubbles in syringe, low hemoglobin level, hemolysis of sample

Nursing Implementation

• *Pretest*

Before a radial artery puncture is executed or a radial arterial line is inserted, perform an Allen's test to ensure adequate collateral circulation to the hand. With the Allen's test, occlude the radial and ulnar arteries with the fingertips while instructing the patient to tighten the fist. Ask the patient to open the fist and remove pressure from the ulnar artery while maintaining pressure on the radial artery. If color returns to the palm and fingers within 5 seconds, there is adequate ulnar circulation.

Prepare ice and heparinized syringe.

✓ QUALITY CONTROL
Excessive amounts of heparin or an air bubble in the syringe will cause inaccurate results. Draw 1 ml of heparin up into a 5- to 10-ml glass syringe or plastic syringe with vented plunger. The plunger is pulled back to coat the barrel of the syringe. Excess heparin is discarded, leaving the needle full of heparin. A 22- or 25-gauge needle is used.

✓ QUALITY CONTROL
The patient's temperature affects results because the ABG machines are calibrated using gases at 37° C. Note on the requisition slip the patient's temperature at the time the blood is drawn.

Instruct the patient about the arterial puncture; it is painful. If the patient is anxious, hyperventilation may occur, giving false readings because CO_2 will be blown off.

Do not obtain an ABG reading for 20 to 30 minutes after a procedure or event that does not reflect the patient's current status (e.g., suctioning).

• During the Test

Nurses in specialized units perform arterial punctures.

The procedure is usually performed by a physician or a respiratory therapist.

If a radial artery is used, the wrist is hyperextended and the arm is externally rotated.

Palpate the artery for the point of maximal impulse.

Cleanse the site with an alcohol swab.

The needle is inserted at a 45- to 90-degree angle at the point of maximal pulsation.

Observe the syringe; the plunger will move upward under arterial pressure.

Withdraw the needle and cork the syringe with the airtight rubber stopper.

Roll the syringe between your palms to mix the blood with the heparin.

Label the syringe and place it on ice.

Send the specimen to the laboratory immediately with a requisition slip marked with the patient's temperature, the Fio_2 value, and the time.

• Posttest

Immediately after the needle is withdrawn, exert pressure on the arterial site for a minimum of 5 minutes. If the patient is taking anticoagulants, pressure on the site should be maintained for at least 10 minutes.

✪ **COMPLICATION ALERT** ✪ Complications from ABG determination result from the trauma of arterial puncture. They include arterial occlusion from hematoma formation or thrombosis, bleeding, and infection. It is essential that the pressure on the artery after the arterial puncture be maintained for a *clocked* 5 minutes.

ARTHROSCOPY • ENDOSCOPY

Synonyms: None

NORMAL VALUES

No tissue or structural abnormalities of the joint space are noted.

Purpose of the Test

Arthroscopy provides direct visualization of the interior of the joint and tissue surfaces. It is used to detect torn ligament, injured meniscus, and damaged cartilage.

Procedure

Two surgical incisions are made in the skin. A trocar is inserted into the joint capsule through one incision, followed by the insertion of the arthroscope. A probe or the accessory instruments are inserted through the other incision. The joint capsule is filled and distended with saline or Ringer's lactate to promote visualization. Additional incisions may be needed to visualize all aspects of the joint. Tissue and fluid samples may be collected for laboratory analysis. Once the fluid is drained and the instruments removed, sutures or tape strips are used to close the incisions. The total time needed for the procedure is 2 to 3 hours.

Diagnostic arthroscopy is performed as a same-day surgical procedure. Either local or general anesthesia may be used. Arthroscopy is an invasive procedure because surgical openings are made into the joint capsule to allow the insertion of the endoscope. Following the diagnostic phase, arthroscopic surgical repair of the torn or damaged tissue may be performed.

Findings

Torn anterior cruciate or tibial collateral ligaments of the knee
Torn medial or lateral meniscus of the knee
Degenerative articular cartilage
Synovitis
Loose bodies
Subluxation, fracture, or dislocation of the bone
Chondromalacia
Osteochondritis dissecans
Arthritis
Gout or pseudogout
Ganglion or Baker's cyst

Interfering Factors

Failure to maintain a nothing-by-mouth status

Nursing Implementation

• *Pretest*

Explain the procedure and obtain a written consent from the patient or person legally designated to make health care decisions for the patient.
Instruct the patient to discontinue all food and fluids for 8 hours before the procedure.
Give instructions for the patient to have a responsible person available to provide transportation after the procedure.
Take baseline vital signs and record the results.

• *Posttest*

If general anesthesia has been administered, take vital signs immediately and thereafter every 15 minutes for 2 hours, every 30 minutes for 1 hour, and every hour for 2 hours or until discharge from the postanesthesia unit.
If local anesthesia has been administered, take initial vital signs and repeat them at regular intervals thereafter.
Assess for pain and provide the prescribed medication for relief of pain, as needed.
Check the elastic compression dressing for any signs of exces-

sive bleeding, constriction, or excessive swelling of the joint or distal extremity.

Inform the patient that walking is permitted, but there should be no exercise or excessive use of the joint for 24 hours.

Provide the prescriptions for medications to be taken at home. Pain is usually minimal and can be relieved by nonsteroidal, anti-inflammatory medications and nonnarcotic analgesics.

✪ **COMPLICATION ALERT** ✪ Since arthroscopy is usually done as a same-day surgery procedure, the nurse needs to educate the patient on how to identify infection of the joint, which is its potential complication. Instruct the patient to report fever, joint swelling, increasing pain, and any purulent, malodorous drainage.

ASPARTATE AMINOTRANSFERASE (AST) • SERUM

NORMAL VALUES

Adult (average range): 8–20 U/L or SI 0.14–0.34 µKat/L
Infant: 15–60 U/L or SI 0.14–0.34 µKat/L
Newborn: 25–75 U/L or SI 0.43–1.28 µKat/L

Purpose of the Test

Aspartate aminotransferase is used to identify inflammation, injury, or necrosis in liver tissue. In liver disease, it is an indicator of hepatocellular damage from any cause. AST is also used to monitor liver function in patients who receive medication that is potentially hepatotoxic.

Procedure

A red-topped sterile tube is used to collect 5 to 10 ml of venous blood.

✓ QUALITY CONTROL
To prevent hemolysis, venipuncture technique must be smooth, with blood flow that fills the tube readily.

Findings

Increase

Hepatitis
Cirrhosis
Hepatic tumor
Obstructive jaundice

Interfering Factors

Hemolysis
Failure to maintain NPO status
Severe exercise prior to the test

Nursing Implementation

- *Pretest*

Instruct the patient to fast for 12 hours before the test (overnight).

The ambulatory patient should avoid strenuous exercise before the test.

- *Posttest*

If the patient is receiving potentially hepatotoxic medication and the AST value rises to three times the upper limit of normal, notify the physician of the elevated test result. This is generally the parameter to discontinue the medication.

B

NORMAL VALUES

No lesions, deficits, or abnormalities of the colon are noted.

Purpose of the Test

The barium enema is used to investigate pathologic changes in the structure or function of the colon.

Procedure

After the colon is completely emptied of feces, the barium is instilled. After the contrast material flows through the entire colon, x-ray images are taken to identify the abnormalities.

Findings

Carcinoma
Diverticulitis
Hirschsprung's disease
Idiopathic megacolon
Polyps
Gastroenteritis
Chronic amebic dysentery
Ulcerative colitis
Crohn's disease
Intussusception

Interfering Factors

Residual barium from an upper GI series
Inability to retain barium
Incomplete cleansing of the colon

Nursing Implementation

• *Pretest*

Schedule this test before any other barium studies.

Provide a complete explanation (verbal and written) of the
procedure for bowel cleansing.

Obtain a signed consent.

Bowel preparation: A clear liquid diet begins 12 to 24
hours before the test. A cathartic (castor oil, magnesium
citrate, or senna extract [X-Prep]) is taken on the afternoon before the test. Bisacodyl (Dulcolax) tablets are
taken on the evening before the test and a bisacodyl
(Dulcolax) suppository is inserted on the morning of the
test. A warm tap water enema (2 L for adults) is given
on the night before the test or at 6 a.m. on the day of
the test. When all fecal matter has been removed, the enema returns will be clear. For children younger than 4
years, the bowel preparation is prescribed on an individualized basis.

Extra oral fluids are taken in the afternoon and evening of the
pretest period to prevent dehydration. Some protocols require a nothing-by-mouth status after midnight.

✓ QUALITY CONTROL

To obtain a clear and accurate visualization of the lumen, all fecal matter, residual gas, and mucus must be removed.

• *Posttest*

The patient is assisted to the toilet to evacuate the contrast medium.

A laxative is prescribed to eliminate the residual barium and
to prevent constipation. Residual barium changes the feces
to a gray or whitish color for 24 to 72 hours.

Encourage the patient to rest for the remainder of the day.
Elderly patients are vulnerable to weakness and may experience a fall. Because they may be dehydrated and
mentally confused, an increase in fluid intake is important.

BILIRUBIN · SERUM

N O R M A L   V A L U E S

TOTAL BILIRUBIN
Adult: 0.3–1 mg/dl *or* SI 5–17 µmol/L
Child: 0.2–0.8 mg/dl *or* SI 3.4–13.6 µmol/L
Full-term neonate: 6–10.0 mg/dl *or* SI 103–171 µmol/L
Premature neonate: 12 mg/dl *or* SI <205 µmol/L

DIRECT BILIRUBIN
Adult: 0.0–0.4 mg/dl *or* SI <5 µmol/L

INDIRECT BILIRUBIN
Adult: 0.2–0.8 mg/dl *or* SI 3.4–13.6 µmol/L

Purpose of the Test

The *total* bilirubin test is used to evaluate liver function, diagnose or monitor the progression of jaundice, and determine whether an infant needs treatment of the jaundice to prevent kernicterus. *Indirect* and *direct* bilirubin tests help identify the underlying cause of hyperbilirubinemia.

Procedure

Adult. A red-topped sterile tube is used to collect 5 to 10 ml of venous blood.

Infants and Neonates. A blue capillary tube is used to draw drops of blood from the heel that has been pricked by a sterile lancet.

✓ QUALITY CONTROL
To prevent hemolysis, venipuncture technique must be smooth, with a blood flow that fills the vacutainer readily.

Findings

Increase

Total serum bilirubin
Hepatocellular damage

Cancer of the liver
Obstruction in the biliary tree
Neonatal (physiologic) jaundice
Hemolytic diseases
Direct bilirubin
Hepatocellular necrosis
Infection in the liver
Cancer of the liver, biliary duct, or pancreas
Cirrhosis
Biliary atresia
Gallstone
Acute pancreatitis
Indirect bilirubin
Hemolytic anemias
Malaria
Hodgkin's disease
Neonatal (physiologic) jaundice
Rh or ABO incompatibility
Blood transfusion reaction

Interfering Factors

Sunlight
Hemolysis
Failure to maintain nothing-by-mouth status (adults only)

Nursing Implementation

• *Pretest*

Instruct the patient to fast from food for 8 to 12 hours because serum lipids would alter results.

• *Posttest*

Insure that the vial of blood or microcapillary tube is covered and sent to the laboratory without delay.

✓ QUALITY CONTROL
Since bilirubin is photosensitive, the blood sample must be protected from exposure to light.

BLOOD CULTURE • BLOOD

N O R M A L   V A L U E S

Negative; no growth of organisms

Purpose of the Test

The blood culture confirms the presence of septicemia, an infection in the blood stream and identifies the causative organism. Susceptibility testing measures the sensitivity of the pathogen to various antibiotics.

Procedure

For the adult, a needle and syringe, a transfer set, or a special set of blood tubes with culture media is used to collect 20 ml of venous blood.

For neonates, infants, and small children, 0.1 to 1 ml of venous blood is obtained for each blood culture specimen. From 1 to 5 ml of blood may be obtained from older children, based on the larger body size and blood volume.

> ✓ QUALITY CONTROL
> The tourniquet should be tied lightly for a brief time to prevent pooling of cells in the vein at the site of blood collection. To prevent hemolysis, venipuncture technique must be smooth, with a blood flow that fills the syringe or tube readily.

Findings

Positive

Septicemia
Bacterial endocarditis
Bacterial meningitis
Typhoid fever
Toxic shock syndrome
Osteomyelitis
Bacterial pneumonia

Interfering Factors

Contamination of the specimen
Hemolysis
Antibiotic therapy

Nursing Implementation

• *Pretest*

Inform the patient about the procedure, including the series
   of blood specimens and skin asepsis.
Ask the patient about skin sensitivity to iodine.
Schedule the tests before antibiotic therapy is started.
To assist with the timing of the blood sampling, monitor the
   patient's temperature, pulse, respirations, and blood pressure at frequent and regular intervals. Record the results.

• *During the Test*

The skin is cleansed at the venipuncture site. The first scrub is
   in concentric circles and in an outward direction with 70%
   alcohol. After it is dry, follow with a second scrub in the
   same pattern using povidone-iodine solution. This dries on
   the skin for at least 1 minute.
The tops of the culture bottles or tubes are cleansed with alcohol or povidone-iodine. Alcohol is used to wipe the stoppers
   of a blood collection system.
Using gloves and aseptic technique, the blood is drawn from
   the vein and then divided among the specimen bottles or
   tubes.

✓ QUALITY CONTROL
If there is an intravenous catheter in place, the specimen is obtained from a venous site below the catheter or from the opposite extremity. The blood cannot be drawn from an intravenous
line or heparin-lock device.

• *Posttest*

Ensure that each requisition slip and all collection containers
   are correctly identified, including the time, date, and venous
   site. Record this same information in the patient's chart.

Arrange for prompt transport of the specimens to the laboratory.

BONE BIOPSY • TISSUE BIOPSY

Synonym: Bone needle aspiration cytology

NORMAL VALUES

Bone tissue is normal with no tumor cells present.

Purpose of the Test

Bone biopsy is performed to examine a specimen of bone tissue for its cell type and to distinguish benign from malignant bone tumor.

Procedure

With local anesthesia, a small incision is made in the skin, and a bone biopsy needle is drilled or pushed into the bone. Once it is in place, the biopsy needle is rotated 180 degrees to obtain a core sample of the tissue. The specimen is placed on a slide with fixative or in a specimen jar with 95% alcohol as a fixative, or both procedures are carried out. The time needed for this procedure is 30 minutes or more.

Findings

Malignancies

Osteogenic sarcoma
Ewing's sarcoma
Reticulum cell sarcoma
Angiosarcoma
Multiple myeloma
Metastatic tumor

Benign tumors

Giant cell tumor
Osteoma
Osteoid osteoma
Chondroma

Interfering Factors

Failure to obtain an adequate sample of tissue
Failure to send the specimen to the laboratory immediately

Nursing Implementation

- ### Pretest

Explain the procedure to the patient and obtain written consent from the patient or person legally designated to make the patient's health care decisions.

Instruct the patient to remove all clothing and put on a hospital gown.

Take baseline vital signs and record the results.

Shave the skin at the biopsy location and cleanse it with antiseptic.

- ### During the Test

Provide support to the patient as the skin and subcutaneous tissue are anesthetized and as the biopsy needle is inserted.

Despite the local anesthetic, momentary pain is experienced as the needle penetrates the periosteum and enters the bone.

Label all specimen containers and slides with the patient's name and the tissue source.

Complete the requisition form for a tissue cytologic study. The requisition slip states the patient's name, age, any history of carcinoma or infection, and the site of biopsy.

Send the slides or specimen, or both, to the laboratory without delay.

✓ QUALITY CONTROL

The final preparation of the slides must be performed within 6 hours to prevent deterioration of the tissue.

- ### Posttest

Take vital signs and monitor them at regular intervals until they are stable.

Determine that the adhesive bandage is clean, dry, and intact.

Observe site for infection. Instruct the patient to notify the physician if untoward symptoms occur.

BONE MARROW EXAMINATION   • MICROSCOPY

N O R M A L   V A L U E S

Normal bone marrow

Purpose of the Test

The bone marrow aspiration and biopsy is used to evaluate hematopoiesis. It diagnoses malignancy of primary and metastatic origin and determines the cause of infection. This examination also is used to evaluate the progression of some hematologic diseases or the response of the marrow to chemotherapy treatment.

Procedure

Using a local anesthetic, a bone marrow needle is inserted into the medullary cavity of a bone. Fluid and marrow cells are aspirated into a glass syringe. A core of marrow tissue may also be removed. Slide specimens of the tissue are prepared and culture specimens may be obtained.

Findings

Anemia (iron deficiency, sideroblastic, megaloblastic, aplastic)
Leukemia
Multiple myeloma
Hodgkin's disease
Lymphoma
Metastatic bone cancer
Macroglobulinemia
Agammaglobulinemia
Myelofibrosis
Collagen disease
Infection

Interfering Factors

Failure to obtain an adequate specimen

Nursing Implementation

- *Pretest*

Assess the patient for the need for additional information or anxiety. Anxiety may be related to fear of the procedure and the possible diagnosis.
Obtain a signed consent.

- *During the Test*

Position the patient according to the site that will be biopsied (sternum, iliac crest, tibia, vertebrae).

Cleanse the skin with an antiseptic solution.

Provide support and reassurance as the local anesthetic is instilled.

Caution the patient to remain immobile as the biopsy needle is inserted into the marrow. Some pain is felt as the marrow is aspirated.

Assist with the preparation and labeling of the slides. The biopsy tissue is placed in a sterile specimen jar that contains a fixative solution.

Once the needle is removed, apply pressure to the site, using a small sterile gauze. Then apply a small sterile dressing.

- *Posttest*

Arrange for prompt transport of the specimens and slides to the laboratory.

Reassure the patient that mild discomfort at the biopsy site is temporary. Persistent bleeding or infection, however, should be reported to the physician.

BREAST BIOPSY • PATHOLOGY

NORMAL VALUES

No malignant cells are seen.

Purpose of the Test

When there is a suspicious palpable or nonpalpable lesion of the breast, a biopsy is used to determine the cause of the lesion and differentiate between benign and malignant tissue.

Procedure

Fluid or tissue is removed from the breast lesion by needle aspiration or surgical excision. Before the surgical biopsy is performed, a needle and a localizing wire are placed into the suspicious tissue, as guided by mammography, ultrasound, or stereotactic measurement. The wire remains in place to help locate the biopsy site and is then removed. Slides of the fluid and tissue are prepared for microscopic examination.

Findings

Fibroadenoma
Carcinoma
Abscess
Duct papilloma
Mastitis
Lipoma
Calcification

Interfering Factors

Inadequate tissue sample

Nursing Implementation

● *Pretest*

Obtain a written consent for the procedure.
If general anesthesia is planned, instruct the patient to fast from food and liquids for 8 hours.
Assess and record the vital signs.
The patient usually experiences a high level of stress, with feelings of anxiety or depression.
Provide emotional support through personalization of the nursing care.

● *During the Test*

Clean the skin with povidone-iodine and apply the sterile drape over the correct breast.
Once the tissue is obtained, place the specimen in a sterile, dry, labeled container. Place the container on ice and arrange for immediate transport of the specimen to the laboratory.
When microscopic slides are prepared, the aspirated material is used to prepare two to four slides. The smears are fixed immediately with 95% alcohol or a spray-on cytologic fixative. The slides are then transported to the laboratory within minutes.
Apply a dry, sterile dressing to the incision or puncture site.

• *Posttest*

Take vital signs and record the results.

With general anesthesia, monitor the vital signs every 15 to 30 minutes until results are stable.

Discharge instructions include avoidance of vigorous exercise for 2 weeks and the use of warm, moist compresses and a supportive bra to relieve pain. The surgical dressing is changed once a day.

Advise the patient to inform the surgeon of redness, swelling, drainage, or excessive pain.

✪ **COMPLICATION ALERT** ✪ Because cellulitis and hematoma can occur, the nurse instructs the patient to report general complaints of fever or headache and the specific breast problems of redness, swelling, pain, bruising, or leakage of blood.

BRONCHOSCOPY • ENDOSCOPY

Synonyms: None

NORMAL VALUES

No abnormalities visualized.
No growth in culture specimen.

Purpose of the Test

Bronchoscopy may be performed for therapeutic or diagnostic purposes. Bronchoscopy is used diagnostically to visualize possible tumors, obstructions, secretions, bleeding sites, or foreign objects in the tracheobronchial system. It permits the collection of secretions for cytologic and bacteriologic study as well as for assessing tumors for potential resection. Tissue for lung biopsy may be obtained through the bronchoscope (transbronchial lung biopsy). A *transcatheter bronchial brushing* may also be carried out to obtain a biopsy. A small brush is inserted through the bronchoscope, which is moved back and forth until cells adhere to the brush. Once the brush is removed, the cells are brushed onto slides.

Bronchoscopy is used therapeutically to remove foreign objects from the tracheobronchial tree and to remove secretions that are obstructing the air passages. A bronchoscope may be used to fulgurate (electrodesiccate) and excise lesions.

Procedure

A rigid (metal) or flexible fiberoptic bronchoscope may be used. The rigid bronchoscope employs a hollow metallic tube with a light at its distal end. It is useful in removing secretions, in evaluating future surgical interventions, and in dilating endobronchial strictures. The rigid bronchoscope has almost been replaced by the flexible fiberoptic bronchoscope. However, the physician may prefer the metal scope under certain circumstances, such as endobronchial tumor resection, massive hemorrhage, foreign body removal, and in the treatment of small children.

The bronchoscope is inserted through the nose (most common) or through the mouth. The tube is inserted as the physician observes the condition of the upper airways through the eyepiece and guides the tube to the area of the lung to be evaluated (Fig. 1 on p. 48).

Findings

Atelectasis
Bleeding
Foreign objects
Infection
Lung cancer
Secretions
Tuberculosis
Tumors

Interfering Factors

Patient distress (may require general anesthesia)

Nursing Implementation

- *Pretest*

Ensure that a signed consent form has been obtained.
Obtain a medication history to determine whether the patient is on anticoagulant therapy or aspirin preparations.
If a prothrombin time (PT), a partial thromboplastin time (PTT), and a platelet count were ordered, check the results and report any clotting problems to the physician.

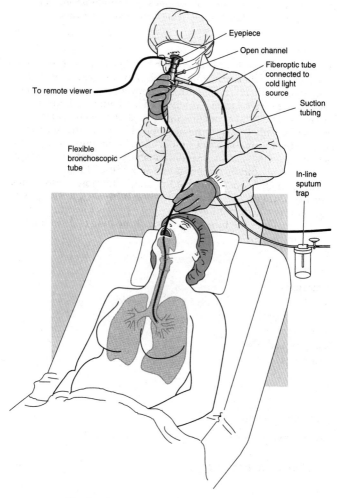

Figure 1. Flexible Fiberoptic Bronchoscopy.

Instruct the patient not to eat or drink for 4 to 6 hours before the test.

Explain the purpose of and procedure for the test.

Warn the patient that the local anesthetic may taste bitter.

Inform the patient that as the tube is inserted it may feel like something is caught in the throat; provide reassurance that the airway is not blocked.

Administer atropine as prescribed to reduce tracheobronchial secretions and inhibit vagal stimulation. A sedative, such as midazolam hydrochloride (Versed), may also be ordered and given. Codeine may be ordered and administered to decrease the cough reflex.

• *During the Test*

The patient is positioned in the semi-Fowler's or Fowler's position.

Attach the patient to the pulse oximeter.

A local anesthetic is sprayed onto the pharynx, and the solution is dropped onto the vocal cords, epiglottis, and trachea to abolish the gag reflex.

Provide the patient with emotional support.

Encourage the patient to breathe through the nose or to pant.

Maintain supplemental O_2 for nonintubated patients.

Continuously monitor the patient's response, vital signs, and Sao_2.

• *Posttest*

Withhold food and fluids until the gag reflex returns.

Reassure the patient that hoarseness, sore throat, and blood-streaked sputum are common.

Provide throat lozenges or throat sprays as comfort measures.

If a biopsy has been performed, send the specimen to the histology laboratory and the microbiology laboratory.

Observe for bleeding, bronchospasms, laryngospasm, and pneumothorax.

⊘ **COMPLICATION ALERT** ⊘ When assessing for pneumothorax following a bronchoscopy, the nurse observes for a mediastinal shift toward the unaffected side. This is indicative of a tension pneumothorax. Observe for tracheal deviation toward the unaffected side and absent or decreased breath sounds over the affected side.

C

CALCITONIN • SERUM, PLASMA

Synonyms: CT, thyrocalcitonin

N O R M A L   V A L U E S

SERUM
Adult male: <40 pg/ml *or* SI <40 ng/L
Adult female: <25 pg/ml *or* SI <25 ng/L
Infant
Cord blood: 30–240 pg/ml *or* SI 30–240 ng/L
7 days old: 77–293 pg/ml *or* SI 77–293 ng/L

PLASMA
Male: ≤19 pg/ml *or* SI ≤19 ng/L
Female: ≤14 pg/ml *or* SI ≤14 ng/L

Purpose of the Test

Calcitonin is a hormone produced and secreted by the parafolli-cular cells (C cells) of the thyroid gland. It may also be produced and secreted by ectopic sites such as the lungs, intestines, pituitary gland, and bladder. The action of calcitonin is to inhibit bone reabsorption, inhibit calcium absorption in the gastrointestinal tract, and increase calcium and phosphate excretion from the kidneys. It is believed that calcitonin is not secreted until plasma calcium levels reach 9.3 ng/dl.

A calcitonin determination is usually performed to diagnose medullary carcinoma of the thyroid gland.

Procedure

Venipuncture is performed to obtain 3 ml venous blood in a hep-arinized green-topped tube. Calcitonin is measured using RIA. To assess familial medullary cancer in relatives of patients with the cancer, a provocation test may be performed. Calcium chloride, 150 mg, is given intravenously over 10 minutes or pentagastrin, 0.5 mg, is given intravenously over 5 to 10 minutes. Patients with medullary cancer will respond to these stimulants with excessive secretion of calcitonin.

Findings

Increase

Cancer of the thyroid
Chronic renal failure
Ectopic secretion by malignant tumors
Endocrine tumors of the pancreas
Pernicious anemia
Subacute Hashimoto's thyroiditis
Parathyroid adenoma or hyperplasia
Pregnancy

Interfering Factors

Noncompliance with fasting requirement

Nursing Implementation

Nursing actions are similar to those in other venipuncture procedures.

- *Pretest*

Instruct the patient not to eat or drink anything but sips of water for 8 hours before the blood is drawn.

- *Posttest*

Inform the laboratory personnel that a calcitonin level is being obtained, as the blood sample must be separated immediately.
The blood sample must be sent to the laboratory immediately after it is drawn.
The patient may resume a normal diet.

CALCIUM • SERUM, URINE

Synonyms: Ca, total serum calcium

NORMAL VALUES

SERUM
Adult: 8.2–10.2 mg/dl *or* SI 2.05–2.54 µmol/L
Infant–1 month: 7–11.5 mg/dl *or* SI 1.75–2.87 µmol/L
Child, 1 month–1 year: 8.6–11.2 mg/dl *or* SI 2.15–2.79 µmol/L

URINE
Adult (normal calcium intake): 100–300 mg/day *or* SI 2.5–7.5 µmol/day
Adult (low calcium intake): 50–100 mg/day *or* SI 1.25–3.75 µmol/day
Adult (calcium-free diet): 5–40 mg/day *or* SI 0.13–1 µmol/day
Infant and child: <6 mg/kg/day *or* SI <0.15 µmol/kg/day

Purpose of the Test

The serum and urine calcium levels are measured to assist in the diagnosis of acid-base imbalance, coagulation disorders, pathologic bone disorders, endocrine disorders, cardiac arrhythmia, and muscle disorders. Excessive calcium in the urine may cause urinary calculi. The most common calcium stones are composed of calcium oxalate and a few are composed of calcium phosphate.

Procedure

Serum

Adult. A red-topped tube is used to collect 1 ml of venous blood.

Infant. A capillary pipette is used to collect capillary blood via the heelstick method.

✓ QUALITY CONTROL
The tourniquet is applied briefly. Venipuncture technique must be smooth, with a flow of blood that fills the vacuum tube readily. If there is venous stasis and pooling or excessive hemolysis, the serum calcium level will be falsely elevated.

Urine

Urine is collected for 24 hours and stored in a clean plastic container or a special glass container that is acid-washed prior to use.

Findings

Increase (hypercalcemia)	*Decrease (hypocalcemia)*
Hyperparathyroidism	Hypoparathyroidism
Polycythemia vera	Acute pancreatitis

Metastatic cancer
Pheochromocytoma
Multiple myeloma
Sarcoidosis
Vitamin D intoxication
Adrenal insufficiency
Milk-alkali syndrome
Thyrotoxicosis
Overuse of calcium antacids
Bacteremia
Paget's disease
Dehydration
Idiopathic hypercalcemia of
   infancy

Vitamin D deficiency
Anterior pituitary hypofunc-
   tion
Chronic renal failure
Alcoholism
Renal tubular disease
Hypoalbuminemia
Cirrhosis of the liver
Massive blood transfusions
Malnutrition
Prolonged intravenous fluid
   therapy
Neonatal prematurity

Interfering Factors

Serum

Upright position or pro-
   longed activity before the
   test
Venous stasis or hemolysis
   during the blood collection
   procedure
Prolonged storage of the
   blood specimen

Urine

Failure to collect all urine in
   the 24-hour collection period

Nursing Implementation

• *Pretest*

Serum

Instruct the patient to fast from food for 8 hours and arrange
   to have the blood drawn in the early morning.
Some medications (i.e., thiazides and other diuretics, lithium,
   and calcium salts) cause a rise in the serum value and may
   be withheld during the period in which the patient ingests
   nothing by mouth, as prescribed.

• *Posttest*

Serum

Arrange for prompt transport of the specimen to the laboratory.

✓ QUALITY CONTROL

The blood specimen may require refrigeration in the laboratory, but the analysis must be performed on a fresh sample. Prolonged storage or a delay in performing the analysis results in a false elevation of the calcium value.

• *Pretest*

Urine

If the test is used to evaluate nephrolithiasis, instruct the patient to eat the usual diet for 3 days before the test. If the patient is already receiving a calcium-restricted diet as part of the calcium stone prevention treatment, instruct the patient to maintain the dietary restriction before and during the test period.

When thiazide diuretics are used to prevent formation of calcium stones, instruct the patient to continue the medication before and during the test. Thiazides are effective in lowering the urine calcium levels, and the benefits of the medication can be evaluated.

Instruct the patient to void at 8 a.m. and discard the specimen.

For 24 hours thereafter, all urine is collected and placed in the large collection container. The 8 a.m. specimen of the following day is included in the collection period.

• *Posttest*

Urine

No special nursing implementation is needed.

| CALCIUM, IONIZED | • SERUM |

Synonyms: Dialyzable calcium, free calcium

N O R M A L   V A L U E S

45–55% of total serum calcium *or* SI 0.45–0.55 (fraction of total serum calcium)

SERUM
Adult: 4.65–5.28 mg/dl *or* SI 1.1–61.32 μmol/L
Child: 4.80–5.52 mg/dl *or* SI 1.20–1.38 μmol/L

Purpose of the Test

Serum calcium levels consist of ionized or free calcium and calcium bound to protein. It is the free calcium that is used by the body. Total calcium levels are influenced by serum albumin levels, but ionized calcium levels are not.

This test is used to assess primary hyperparathyroidism, especially in patients with low albumin levels.

Procedure

Venipuncture is performed to fill a red-topped tube. Exposure to air is prevented by using a vacuum tube.

Findings

Since ionized calcium in blood increases and decreases with blood pH, any condition that causes a variation in the blood pH will cause a change in the free calcium level. The following, therefore, is a partial listing.

Increase	*Decrease*
Acidosis	Alkalosis
Acromegaly	Acute pancreatitis
Addison's disease	Diarrhea
Ectopic neoplasms	Hypomagnesemia
Hyperparathyroidism	Hypoparathyroidism
Prolonged immobility	Malabsorption
Osteoporosis	Multiple blood transfusions
Paget's disease	Osteomalacia
Pheochromocytoma	Renal failure
	Starvation
	Vitamin D deficiency

Interfering Factors

Diet high in calcium

Diet deficient in vitamin D

Multiple drugs (including antacids, anticonvulsants, aspirin, barbiturates, gentamicin, insulin, lithium, steroids, thiazide diuretics, thyroid hormones)

Nursing Implementation

The nurse provides actions similar to those of other venipuncture techniques.

• Pretest

The patient maintains bed rest in a supine position for 30 minutes before the blood is drawn.

• Posttest

Refrigerate specimen or send to the laboratory on ice immediately.

CANCER ANTIGEN 125 (CA 125)	• SERUM, BODY FLUID

N O R M A L   V A L U E S
<35 U/ml *or* SI <35 kU/L

Purpose of the Test

Cancer antigen 125 is a tumor marker for ovarian cancer. The test is used to monitor the progress of disease in the patient after the surgical removal of the tumor. The analysis of body fluids for cancer antigen 125 helps diagnose malignancy of an organ in the body cavity.

Procedure

Serum

A red-topped tube with a serum separator is used to collect 7 ml of venous blood.

Body Fluid

During thoracentesis or paracentesis aspiration, a sample of the body fluid is collected in three sterile tubes (red, green, and lavender tops).

Findings

Increase

Ovarian cancer

Adenocarcinoma (cervix, endometrium, fallopian tubes, lung, colon, pancreas, or breast)

Interfering Factors

Inadequate specimen identification

Recent radioactive isotope scan

Nursing Implementation

- *Pretest*

Schedule this test before or at least 7 days after any radioimmunoassay scan. The radioisotopes of the scan would interfere with the radioimmunoassay method of analysis.

If thoracentesis or paracentesis is performed to obtain a sample of body fluid, the nursing care is presented in the text sections for those procedures.

For the patient with a history of cancer, provide empathetic support. Her anxiety level is likely to be high because of the implications of a potentially elevated or rising test value.

- *Posttest*

Insure that the specimen tubes are correctly identified. The source of the body fluid (thoracentesis or paracentesis fluid) is written on the requisition slip.

Arrange for prompt transport of the specimen to the laboratory.

✓ QUALITY CONTROL

The serum must be separated from the cells quickly. It is frozen until it can be analyzed.

CAPNOGRAM

Synonyms: Exhaled carbon dioxide, capnography, end-tidal carbon dioxide ($ETCO_2$), $Petco_2$

NORMAL VALUES

35–45 mm Hg

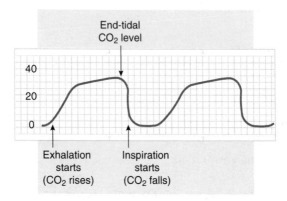

Figure 2. Capnograph Tracing. On exhalation the capnograph tracing shows a rapid rise in carbon dioxide followed by a plateau. At the end of exhalation, the end-tidal carbon dioxide level is obtained. As inspiration begins, there is a dramatic decrease in carbon dioxide.

Purpose of the Test

Monitoring exhaled CO_2 permits continuous evaluation of alveolar ventilation, reducing the number of ABG determinations needed. $Petco_2$ can be used to evaluate ventilator changes and weaning parameters from mechanical ventilation. It will confirm endotracheal intubation, since no capnographic waveform will occur if the tube is in the esophagus. $Petco_2$ is also used to assess the adequacy of cardiopulmonary resuscitation.

Carbon dioxide is measured at the end of exhalation because at this point the exhaled CO_2 approximates arterial CO_2 levels. With normal perfusion of the lungs, arterial CO_2 will be a few millimeters higher (5 mm Hg) than end-tidal CO_2 ($Petco_2$). When perfusion is not adequate, this assumption cannot be made. Figure 2 shows a typical tracing of a capnogram.

Procedure

Exhaled CO_2 is measured with exhaled gas analyzers. These analyzers measure the CO_2 by mass spectrometry or infrared analysis. Mass spectrometry requires aspiration of exhaled gas, whereas the infrared gas analyzer is usually attached to the exhalation tubing on a ventilator. The recorded value refers to the amount of infrared light absorbed by the exhaled breath. The higher the

CO_2 level, the more infrared light absorbed, and the higher the reading.

Findings

Increase	*Decrease*
Burns	Acute cardiac failure
Hypermetabolic states	Anesthesia
Hypoventilation	Bronchial spasms
Malignant hyperthermia	Cardiopulmonary arrest
Multiple trauma	Dislodgment of endotracheal tube
	Hypothermia
	Hypothyroidism
	Hypovolemia
	Leak in mechanical ventilation system
	Pulmonary edema
	Pulmonary embolism

Interfering Factors

Cardiopulmonary abnormalities
Metabolic disorders

Nursing Implementation

- *During the Test*

Check the capnographic waveform. It should return to zero baseline on inspiration. If it does not, check the seal of the expiratory demand valve on the ventilator and the fresh gas flow in the tube.

If the waveform disappears or drops to zero, it may indicate accidental extubation, obstruction, esophageal intubation, or cardiac arrest.

If FiO_2 is greater than .60, accuracy of the capnographic readings is questionable.

CARBOHYDRATE ANTIGEN 19-9 (CA 19-9) • SERUM

N O R M A L   V A L U E S

Adult: <37 U/ml *or* SI <37 kU/L

Purpose of the Test

CA 19-9 is a tumor marker that monitors the course of the disease, the success of therapy and predicts the recurrence of stomach, liver, pancreatic, and colorectal cancer. In benign disease, the serum level is usually <100 U/ml (SI <100 kU/L) but in malignancy the value is much higher.

Procedure

A red-topped tube with a serum separator is used to obtain 5 to 10 ml of venous blood.

Findings

Elevated

Cancer (intraabdominal, pancreas, stomach, liver, biliary system, colon)
Inflammatory bowel disease
Acute pancreatitis
Hepatobiliary disease

Interfering Factors

None

Nursing Implementation

No specific patient instruction or intervention is needed.

CARBON DIOXIDE, TOTAL • SERUM

Synonyms: Carbon dioxide content, Tco_2

N O R M A L   V A L U E S
Adult (venous): 22–26 mEq/L *or* SI 22–26 µmol/L
Adult (arterial): 19–24 mEq/L *or* SI 19–24 µmol/L
Infant (capillary): 20–28 mEq/L *or* SI 20–28 µmol/L

Purpose of the Test

The total carbon dioxide determination is used to help evaluate acid-base balance and the bicarbonate buffer system. It is part of the routine blood chemistry screen or SMA (sequential multiple analyzer).

Procedure

For venous blood testing, a red-capped tube is used to collect 10 ml of venous blood.

For arterial blood testing, a green-topped tube with heparin is used to obtain 5 ml of arterial blood.

For capillary blood testing, a puncture of the heel, earlobe, or finger and a capillary tube are used to collect capillary blood.

✓ QUALITY CONTROL

The rubber stopper must remain firmly in place so that the carbon dioxide cannot diffuse out and result in a falsely lowered value.

Findings

Increase (hypercapnia)

Respiratory acidosis
Metabolic alkalosis
Emphysema
Hypokalemia
Pneumonia
Excessive intake of antacids
Cystic fibrosis
Severe, prolonged vomiting
Congestive heart failure
Cushing's syndrome
Pulmonary edema
Primary aldosteronism

Decrease (hypocapnia)

Respiratory alkalosis
Renal tubular acidosis
Hyperventilation
Renal failure
Metabolic acidosis
Dehydration
Diabetes mellitus
Hypovolemia
Severe diarrhea

Interfering Factors

For venous sampling, none; for arterial sampling see ABGs (p. 28)

Nursing Implementation

No specific patient instruction or intervention is needed.

CARCINOEMBRYONIC ANTIGEN (CEA)	• SERUM, EFFUSION FLUID

NORMAL VALUES

ADULT
Nonsmoker: <2.5 ng/ml *or* SI 2.5 µg/L
Smoker: up to 5 ng/ml *or* SI 5 µg/L

Purpose of the Test

This test is a tumor marker used to (1) monitor the success of cancer therapy, (2) stage colorectal cancer, and (3) monitor for recurrence of cancer in the gastrointestinal tract, particularly colorectal cancer.

Procedure

A red- or lavender-topped tube is used to collect 5 to 10 ml of venous blood. Effusion fluid is collected during a thoracentesis or paracentesis procedure.

✓ QUALITY CONTROL
To prevent hemolysis, venipuncture technique must be smooth, with a blood flow that fills the vacuum tube readily. The serum must be chilled immediately and radioimmunoassay analysis performed within 24 hours.

Findings

Increase

Cancer (colorectal, stomach, pancreas, breast, medullar, thyroid, lung, ovary)
Ulcerative colitis
Chrohn's disease
Hepatitis
Cirrhosis
Pulmonary infection

Interfering Factors

Recent administration of radioisotopes
Smoking
Hemolysis

Nursing Implementation

- *Pretest*

The schedule for testing and monitoring the patient's condition is as follows: presurgery, 4 weeks postoperatively, monthly for 1 to 2 years, and at regular intervals thereafter for a total testing time of 5 years.

Schedule this test before or 7 days after a radioisotope study.

If the patient is a smoker, indicate this information on the requisition slip.

- *Posttest*

The serum sample is packed in a container with ice and is sent directly to the laboratory.

CATECHOLAMINES • PLASMA, URINE

Synonyms: Catecholamine fractionalization, plasma

NORMAL VALUES

SERUM

CATECHOLAMINE	Supine	Standing
Epinephrine:	<50 pg/ml or SI <273 pmol/L	<900 pg/ml or SI <4914 pmol/L
Norepinephrine:	110–410 pg/ml or SI 650–2423 pmol/L	125–700 pg/ml or SI 739–4137 pmol/L
Dopamine:	<87 pg/ml or SI <475 pmol/L	<87 pg/ml or SI <475 pmol/L

URINE

Norepinephrine: <100 ng/d 24 hours or SI <591 nmol/d 24 hours

Epinephrine: <10 ng/d 24 hours or SI <55 nmol/d 24 hours

Dopamine: 65–400 ug/d or SI 384–2364 nmol/d 24 hours

Vanillylmandelic acid: 2–7 mg/24 hours or SI 10–35 µmol/24 hours

Metanephrine: 0.1–1.6 mg/d or SI 0.5–8.7 µmol/d 24 hours

Purpose of the Test

Plasma catecholamines are usually assessed to diagnose pheo-chromocytoma or to identify extraadrenal tumors. Pheochro-mocytomas are tumors developing in the sympathetic nervous system. These tumors usually secrete epinephrine or norepi-nephrine, or both, sometimes dopamine.

Procedure

Serum

Plasma catecholamines are measured using radioenzymatic tech-nique. A venous sampling of 3 ml of blood is drawn into a green-topped tube with ethylenediaminetetraacetic acid (EDTA), once while the patient is lying down and then with the patient stand-ing. The normal values vary among laboratories. Results may not reveal a tumor that secretes intermittently, so the test may be ordered for when the patient is symptomatic. To localize small tumors, percutaneous venous catheterization may be needed.

A *clonidine suppression test* may be performed to differentiate between pheochromocytoma and essential hypertension. With this test, clonidine is given 2 to 3 hours before a venous blood sample is taken. Clonidine suppresses neurogenic catecholamine release. If suppression occurs, the test result is consistent with the diagnosis of essential hypertension. If the catecholamines remain elevated, the diagnosis of pheochromocytoma is supported.

Urine

A 24-hour urine specimen is collected with an acid preservative added to the container.

Findings

Increase

Pheochromocytoma
Ganglioneuroma
Neuroblastoma

Interfering Factors for Plasma Catecholamine Levels

Noncompliance with diet and relaxation requirements
Anger

Severe anxiety
Amine-rich foods and drinks
Cold environment
Medications (amphetamines, barbiturates, decongestants, epi-
    nephrine, levodopa, phenothiazines, reserpine, sympathomi-
    metics, tricyclic antidepressants)

Interfering Factors for Urinary Catecholamines
Note that interfering factors vary with the laboratory technique
used.

Epinephrine:	Stress
Norepinephrine:	Exercise
Dopamine:	Foods and drugs containing catecholamines
	High-fluorescent compounds (e.g., tetracycline and quinidine)
	Levodopa
	Methyldopa
Metanephrine:	Catecholamines and mono-amine oxidase (MAO) inhibitors
Normetanephrine:	Severe stress
Vanillylmandelic acid:	Catecholamines
	Foods with vanilla
	Levodopa
	MAO inhibitors

Nursing Implementation

• *Pretest*

Serum

Instruct the patient to avoid amine-rich foods and drinks for
    48 hours before the test (e.g., avocados, bananas, beer,
    cheese, chianti wine, cocoa, coffee, and tea).
Instruct the patient not to smoke for 24 hours before the
    test.
Explain to the patient that a venous catheter (heparin lock) is

inserted 24 hours before the blood sample is drawn, as venipuncture may increase catecholamine levels.
Instruct the patient to lie down and relax for an hour before
the blood is drawn.

• *During the Test*

Serum

The nurse carries out duties
similar to those of other
venipuncture procedures,
except that blood is drawn
through the heparin lock.
If heparin lock was flushed
with heparin withdraw
approximately 2 to 3 ml
of blood and discard be-
fore obtaining the spec-
imen.

After the first sample is
drawn, the patient stands
for 10 minutes, and a second sample is drawn.

Include on the requisition
slip the position of the patient when the blood was
drawn.

Flush heparin lock according
to hospital protocol.

Urine

At the start of the test, instruct the patient to void
at 8 a.m. and discard this
urine. The collection pe-
riod begins at this time and
all urine is collected for 24
hours, including the 8 a.m.
specimen on the following
morning.

On the requisition slip and
specimen label, write the
patient's name and the
time and date of the start
and finish of the test period.

Keep the urine specimen refrigerated or on ice
throughout the collection
period.

• *Posttest*

Serum

The patient may resume pretest diet and activity. Notify the laboratory that the specimen is coming, since it must be frozen immediately.

Urine

Arrange for prompt transport of the cooled specimen to the laboratory.

CATHETERIZATION, CARDIAC • RADIOLOGY

Synonyms: Angiocardiography, coronary arteriography

NORMAL VALUES

Pressures
  Right atrium: 1–16 mm Hg
    Neonate: 0–3 mm Hg
    Children: 1–5 mm Hg
  Right ventricle: 15–25/0–6 mm Hg
    Neonate: 30–60/2–5 mm Hg
    Children: 15–30/2–5 mm Hg
  Pulmonary artery pressure: 15–25/5–15 mm Hg
    Neonate: 30–60/2–10 mm Hg
    Children: 15–30/5–10 mm Hg
  Pulmonary artery wedge pressure: 6–12 mm Hg
  Left atrium: 4–12 mm Hg
    Neonate: 1–4 mm Hg
    Children: 5–10 mm Hg
  Left ventricle: 90–140/4–12 mm Hg
    Neonate: 60–100/5–10 mm Hg
    Children: 80–130/10–20 mm Hg
Cardiac output: 4–8 L/minute
Cardiac index: 2.5–4 L/minute
  Neonate and children: 3.5–4 L/minute
Stroke index: 30–60 ml/beat/minute
Ejection fraction: 55–75%
Oxygen saturation: 75% (right side of heart)
95% (left side of heart)
Oxygen content: 14–15 vol % (right side of heart)
19 vol % (left side of heart)
Oxygen consumption: 250 ml/minute
Volume
Left ventricular end-diastolic: 50–90 ml
Left ventricular end-systolic: 14–34 ml

Purpose of the Test

Cardiac catheterization is an invasive procedure that permits the assessment of anatomic abnormalities of the heart. Cardiac catheterization may assess (1) pressures, oxygen content, and oxygen saturation in the various heart chambers; (2) cardiac output and index; (3) patency of the coronary arteries; and (4) pressure gradients across the valves.

Cardiac catheterization may be a right-sided catheterization, a left-sided catheterization, or both. A right-sided catheterization is performed today in specialized units under the category of hemodynamic monitoring; therefore, this section will focus on left-sided catheterization.

A cardiac catheterization is performed to (1) evaluate coronary artery disease with unstable, progressive, or new-onset angina or angina that is not responding to medical therapy; (2) diagnose atypical chest pain; (3) diagnose complications of myocardial infarctions such as septal rupture and refractory dysrhythmias; (4) diagnose aortic dissection; (5) evaluate the need for coronary artery surgery or angioplasty; (6) assess valvular function; and (7) determine the efficacy of a heart transplant. Rarely, a cardiac catheterization may be carried out to obtain a biopsy specimen.

Procedure

A left-sided catheterization is performed in a cardiac catheterization laboratory. This laboratory is designed with fluoroscopy, electrocardiographic equipment, and emergency equipment and drugs (code cart). For a left-sided catheterization, a catheter must be threaded through an artery into the left side of the heart; therefore, arterial access is necessary. Pressure measurements are obtained in the aorta and left atrium and ventricle. Samples of blood are obtained for oxygen analysis. Cardiac output, stroke volume, and ejection fractions are measured.

When a *coronary angiogram* is included in the test, dye is instilled into the heart to visualize the size of the ventricles, wall motion, and contractility and to identify valvular dysfunction.

A *coronary arteriogram* may also be obtained. The catheter is withdrawn from the left ventricle and positioned at the coronary ostia, where small boluses of dye are injected into the coronary arteries while a series of x-ray films are taken.

Findings

CAD
Coronary occlusions and degree of blockage
Congenital abnormalities
Septal defects
Shunting
Aneurysms
Valvular defects

Interfering Factors

Allergic reactions to contrast medium
Uncontrolled congestive heart failure
Dysrhythmias
Renal insufficiency
Electrolyte imbalances
Infection
Drug toxicity

Nursing Implementation

• Pretest

Verify that an informed consent has been obtained.

Instruct the patient about the purpose and procedure for the study. Explain to the patient that the table rotates and that the physician may ask the patient to change positions or cough. Explain to the patient when the dye is given, a feeling of warmth, flushing, or metallic taste may be sensed.

Assist with the precatheterization evaluation—blood work, including a prothrombin time and a partial thromboplastin time; an electrocardiogram (ECG); and chest x-ray film if the procedure will be performed on an outpatient basis. Obtain the patient's height and weight.

If contrast dye is going to be used, check for allergies. Report elevated BUN or creatinine levels, as these patients may be at risk for renal failure.

Assess the patient's fears. Correct any misperceptions and reassure the patient that there will be a continuous presence by the nurse, physician, and technicians to assist during the procedure.

The patient is to have nothing-by-mouth after midnight, except if the catherization is planned for late in the afternoon. In that case, a clear liquid breakfast may be taken. Cardiac drugs are usually continued.

Prepare catheter site according to laboratory protocols. The femoral artery is commonly used for the percutaneous insertion of the catheter. Usually both groins are prepared.

Premedication is given as ordered to reduce the patient's anxiety. In some catheterization laboratories, the patient is premedicated to decrease the risk of allergic reaction to the contrast dye.

Encourage the patient to wear glasses, if required, to the catheterization (cath) laboratory.

Patient is instructed to void before going to the cath lab.

• During the Test

The patient is awake. The nurse provides emotional support and reinforces explanations given about the procedure.

Continuous cardiac monitoring is maintained.

A local anesthetic is used after the insertion site is prepared and draped.

The physician inserts the cardiac catheter under fluoroscopy.

The patient may be asked to change position or cough during the procedure.

Observe constantly for complications, especially dysrhythmia from catheter irritation or sensitivity to the contrast dye.

Heparin is usually given during the procedure to prevent emboli. At the end of the procedure, protamine sulfate is given to reverse heparin's effect.

• Posttest

Observe the insertion site for signs of bleeding. Palpate around the puncture site to detect bleeding into tissue. If bleeding is present, exert pressure just proximal to the puncture site with a gloved hand for a minimum of 15 minutes.

Monitor vital signs and cardiac monitor according to hospital protocol.

Check distal pulses for arterial patency every 15 minutes × 4, then every 30 minutes to 1 hour.

Encourage fluid intake as the contrast dye acts as an osmotic diuretic.

Report any significant changes in vital signs, rhythm, and circulation or the occurrence of chest pain.

Evaluate the patient's psychologic response to the procedure and its findings.

Observe for complications: Allergic reaction to the dye, retroperitoneal bleeding, thrombus, emboli, hematoma at insertion site.

✪ **COMPLICATION ALERT** ✪ A feared complication of a cardiac catheterization is a cardiac tamponade. If a tamponade occurs, it is a surgical emergency. Observe for and report *immediately* signs of decreased cardiac output, muffled heart sounds, and decreasing amplitude of QRS complexes.

CEREBROSPINAL FLUID ANALYSIS AND LUMBAR PUNCTURE

• CEREBROSPINAL FLUID

Synonyms: CSF analysis, spinal tap, LP

N O R M A L   V A L U E S

CEREBROSPINAL FLUID ANALYSIS
Pressure: 90–180 mm H_2O (lateral recumbent position)
Appearance: clear, colorless

Microscopic Examination
Leukocyte count
 Adult: 0–5 cells per μl *or* SI 0–5 × 10^6/L
 Child (5–18 years): 0–10 cells per μl *or* SI 0–10 × 10^6/L
 Neonatal year: 0–30 cells per μl *or* SI 0–30 × 10^6/L
Differential count
 Adult
  Lymphoctes: 40–80%
  Monocytes: 15–45%
  Neutrophils: 0–6%
 Neonate
  Lymphocytes: 5–35%
  Monocytes: 50–90%
  Neutrophils: 0–8%

Chemistry Analysis
Lactate: 10–22 mg/dl *or* SI 1.1–2.4 μmol/L
Glucose: 50–80 mg/dl *or* SI 2.75–4.4 μmol/L
Total protein
 Albumin: 15–45 mg/dl *or* SI 150–450 mg/L
 IgG: 10–30 mg/dl *or* SI 100–300 mg/L
Protein electrophoresis (% of total protein)
 Prealbumin: 1–4 mg/dl *or* SI 10–40 mg/L
 Albumin: 2–7%
 Alpha₁-globulin: 56–76%
 Alpha₂-globulin: 2–7%
 Beta globulin: 4–12%

Purpose of the Test

A lumbar puncture is performed to measure the pressure of the cerebrospinal fluid, to detect obstruction in the circulation of this fluid, and to obtain a sample of cerbrospinal fluid (CSF).

Analysis of the cerebrospinal fluid is performed to confirm the diagnosis of infection in the central nervous system, to identify a tumor or hemorrhage in the brain, spinal cord, or surrounding lining of the tissues. It may be performed to confirm a chronic central nervous system infection such as neurosyphilis.

Procedure

Under sterile conditions and using local anesthesia, a spinal needle is inserted by the physician between the lower lumbar vertebrae into the subarachnoid space. Insertion site is usually between L4 and L5, which is below the end of the spinal cord. After pressure measurements, 15 to 20 ml of cerebrospinal fluid is collected in three or more sterile tubes.

If a lumbar puncture cannot be done in the lower spine, because of scarring, blockage of CSF pathway or skin infection, a *cisternal puncture* may be done. A needle is inserted into the cisterna magna at the C1 and C2 level. A cisternal puncture is *not* the procedure of choice, as it has a higher risk for complications.

Findings

Increase

Leukocytes: Bacterial meningitis

Neutrophils: Bacterial meningitis, encephalomyelitis

Lymphocytes: Meningitis, parasitic infection

Plasma cells: Multiple sclerosis, Guillain-Barré syndrome

Malignant cells: Leukemia, lymphoma, medulloblastoma, metastatic carcinoma

Lactate: Low arterial pO_2, hypotension, stroke, hydrocephalus, brain trauma, cerebral edema, meningitis, cerebral arteriosclerosis, cerebral abscess, cerebral hemorrhage, cerebral infarction, tumor

Eosinophils: Parasitic infection, fungal infection, allergic reaction within the central nervous system

Glucose: Hyperglycemia

Total protein: Meningitis, stroke, extradural abscess, endocrine disorder, trauma, tumor, herniated disc, multiple sclerosis, neurosyphilis

Alpha$_2$-globulin: Severe craniocerebral trauma

Gamma globulin: Multiple sclerosis

Oligoclonal bands: Multiple sclerosis, subacute sclerosing panencephalitis, Jakob-Creutzfeldt's disease, encephalitis, Guillain-Barré syndrome, neurosyphilis, cerebrovascular accident, cerebral vasculitis, neoplasm

Albumin: Viral meningitis, Guillain-Barré syndrome, collagen diseases

IgG: Multiple sclerosis, sclerosing panencephalitis, neurosyphilis

Myelin-Basic protein: Multiple sclerosis, head trauma, cerebrovascular accident, leukemia, neurosyphilis, systemic lupus erythematosus, Guillain-Barré syndrome

Decrease

Glucose: Acute, chronic meningitis, meningoencephalitis, systemic hypoglycemia, subarachnoid hemorrhage, neurosyphilis, sarcoidosis (meningeal), carcinomatous meningitis

Total protein: Dural tear from trauma, increased intracranial pressure

Interfering Factors

Infection of skin or epidural abscess at the site of the proposed spinal tap

Increased intracranial pressure

Spinal block (incomplete or complete)

Bleeding disorder

Nursing Implementation

- *Pretest*

Obtain written consent from the patient or the person legally responsible for the patient's health care decisions.

Ask the patient about any history of hemophilia, thrombocytopenia, other bleeding disorder, or anticoagulation therapy. Because these problems will result in prolonged bleeding into the tissues or cerebrospinal fluid, they are a relative contraindication to lumbar puncture.

Assist the patient in removing all clothing and putting on a hospital gown.

Inform the patient that local anesthetic will be used, but a pressure sensation may be felt.

Take and record vital signs.

Place the patient in a lateral recumbent position with his or her back at the edge of the bed or examining table. Flex the patient's neck and knees toward the chest. The flexion of the spine widens the intervertebral spaces.

If the patient cannot be placed in the lateral recumbent position, place them in a sitting position leaning over a bedside table.

⊙ **COMPLICATION ALERT** ⊙ Assess the patient for severe increase in intracranial pressure. If intracranial pressure is very high, a lumbar puncture may cause brain stem herniation.

• *During the Test*

Assist with the preparation of the equipment and sterile field, the antiseptic cleansing of the skin, and the preparation of the local anesthetic. Usually, lidocaine, 1 to 2 ml, is administered subcutaneously by the physician.

Instruct the patient to remain absolutely still during the insertion of each needle. Hold the patient in position to help prevent movement.

Provide reassurance to the patient as the needles are inserted. The administration of the anesthetic may cause a stinging sensation. There is brief pain as the spinal needle penetrates the dura and enters the subarachnoid space.

Assist the patient in placing the legs in extension for the pressure reading. Record pressure readings.

Assist with the collection of the cerebrospinal fluid. Mark the tubes "1, 2, 3," and so on in the order that they are collected.

✓ QUALITY CONTROL
The first tube is used for chemical and immunologic analysis because blood or tissue fluid will not alter these test results. The second tube is used for microbial analysis, and the third tube is used for microscopic examination of cells. If only a small amount of fluid is drawn, it is placed in a single tube and the physician prioritizes the tests.

Arrange for immediate delivery of the specimen to the laboratory.

✓ QUALITY CONTROL

With delay, lysis of the white blood cells results in a false decrease in the cell count. Additionally, glycolysis causes a false rise in the lactate value and the microbial organisms may be destroyed. If there is an unavoidable delay in the laboratory, tube No. 1 (chemical and immunologic tests) is frozen, tube No. 2 (microbiologic tests) is kept at room temperature, and tube No. 3 (cell counts and cytologic study) is refrigerated.

• Posttest

Take vital signs at regular and frequent intervals until they are stable. At the same time, assess the patient's level of consciousness and responsiveness.

Assess the puncture site for swelling, redness, or leakage of cerebrospinal fluid.

Instruct the patient to lie flat in a supine position for 1 to 6 hours. This helps prevent headache following lumbar puncture. If headache occurs, bedrest is extended to 12 hours.

Administer extra fluids to help the patient replace the volume of fluid in the subarachnoid space and to help prevent headache.

Administer the prescribed pain medication, as needed.

At regular intervals, assess the patient's motor ability in the lower legs. If there is spinal blockage and severe compression of the cord following the procedure, paresis can turn into paralysis. In addition, massive hematoma can occur within the subarachnoid space. This would compress the cauda equina and result in paralysis.

CHLORIDE, SERUM   • SERUM

Synonym: Cl⁻

N O R M A L   V A L U E S

Adult and child: 98–107 mEq/L *or* SI 98–107 µmol/L
Newborn: 98–113 mEq/L *or* SI 98–113 µmol/L
Premature: 95–110 mEq/L *or* SI 95–110 µmol/L

Purpose of the Test

Serum chloride measurements are obtained in the evaluation of electrolyte levels, water balance, and acid-base balance and in the measurement of the cation-anion balance (anion gap). It is part of the routine blood chemistry screen or SMA (sequential multiple analyzer).

Procedure

A red-topped tube is used to collect 7 ml of venous blood. In infants, a heelstick, finger, or earlobe puncture and a capillary tube may be used to collect capillary blood.

> ✓ QUALITY CONTROL
> Venipuncture technique must be smooth, with a blood flow that fills the vacuum tube readily. If there is excessive turbulence because of poor technique, the hemolysis of the erythrocytes will alter the test results.

Findings

Increase (hyperchloremia)

Dehydration
Diabetes insipidus
Renal tubular acidosis
Respiratory alkalosis
Prolonged diarrhea
Hyperparathyroidism
Acute renal failure
Adrenocortical hyperfunction

Decrease (hypochloremia)

Prolonged vomiting
Addison's disease
Nasogastric drainage
Congestive heart failure
Salt-losing nephritis
Intestinal fistula
Chronic renal failure
Overhydration
Metabolic alkalosis
Syndrome of inappropriate
    antidiuretic hormone
Chronic respiratory acidosis
Diuretic therapy

Interfering Factors

Hemolysis
Warming of the specimen

Nursing Implementation

• *Pretest*

For a routine test, instruct the patient to discontinue all food and fluids for 8 hours before the test. This prevents the normal drop in value after eating. For tests performed on an urgent or emergency basis, the fasting status is omitted.

● *Posttest*

Arrange for prompt transport of the blood to the laboratory. The serum or plasma will require refrigeration until the analysis can be performed.

COLD STIMULATION TEST ● SKIN TEMPERATURE

Synonym: Cold sensitivity test

N O R M A L   V A L U E S

The temperature in the fingers returns to normal within 15 minutes.

Purpose of the Test

In vasospastic disorders that affect the arterial circulation of the upper extremities, hypersensitivity to cold is a common complaint. In normal circulation, exposure of the hands and fingers to cold causes temporary vasoconstriction and a lowering of the temperature in the fingers. Once the cold temperature source is eliminated, the circulation improves and the temperature of the fingers returns to normal within 15 minutes. Patients with upper extremity vasospastic disorders require a much longer time to recover normal skin temperature, so this test assists in assessing patients with suspected vasospastic disorders.

Procedure

The temperature of the fingers is recorded before and after the hands are immersed in ice water. The total time required for this test is 30 to 60 minutes.

Findings

Raynaud's syndrome
Rheumatoid arthritis
Scleroderma
Systemic lupus erythematosus

Interfering Factors

Nicotine
Caffeine
Excessively warm or cool room temperature
Gangrenous fingers
Open wounds or infection in hands or fingers

Nursing Implementation

- *Pretest*

Instruct the patient to refrain from smoking and ingesting caffeine (cola, cocoa, coffee, tea) for 24 hours before the test because they are vasoconstrictive substances.

Remove any jewelry from the patient's fingers and wrist.

Inform the patient that the ice water can cause some temporary discomfort in the fingers, but it will disappear after the fingers are warm.

- *During the Test*

Apply the thermistors to the distal part of the fingers of both hands. The thermistors record the skin temperature.

Record the baseline thermistor temperature.

Immerse the hands in ice water for 20 seconds.

Record the temperature immediately after removal of the hands from the water.

Record the temperature every 5 minutes until the temperature returns to the pretest baseline value.

- *Posttest*

Remove the thermistors.

COLONOSCOPY (LOWER PANENDOSCOPY)	• ENDOSCOPY

N O R M A L   V A L U E S

No abnormalities of structure or mucosal surface are observed in the colon or terminal ileum.

Purpose of the Test

Colonoscopy is used to identify and biopsy abnormal tissue in the colon and terminal ileum, investigate the cause of chronic diarrhea, locate the source of GI bleeding, and evaluate the colon for recurrent polyps or malignant growth.

Procedure

Using intravenous sedation, the endoscope is inserted into the rectum and passed through the sigmoid, descending, transverse, and ascending colon, cecum, and possibily the distal ileum. The lumen is visualized and tissue specimens may be collected for cytology examination.

Findings

Diverticulitis
Ulcerative colitis
Polyps
Carcinoma
Colitis
"Gay bowel syndrome"
Crohn's disease

Interfering Factors

Massive bleeding
Inflammatory bowel disease
Stricture
Peritonitis
Bowel perforation
Recent acute cardiopulmonary disease
Recent pelvic or colon surgery
Large aortic or iliac aneurysm
Pregnancy, second or third trimester
Uncooperative behavior
Poor bowel preparation
Retained barium
Failure to maintain pretest dietary restrictions

Nursing Implementation

- *Pretest*

Schedule this test before any barium studies.
Obtain a written consent.

Provide instructions about bowel cleansing.

Lengthy preparation: Begin a clear liquid diet 48 hours before the test. Milk of magnesia, 2 oz, is taken 2 nights before the test and magnesium citrate, 10 oz, is taken on the night before the test. A tap water enema is administered on the night before the test and additional tap water enemas are administered at 6 a.m. until the enema returns are clear.

Rapid preparation: Eat a normal breakfast and a light lunch on the day before the test. Clear liquids are then permitted until midnight when the nothing-by-mouth status begins. At 4 p.m. the lavage solution is taken orally. This preparation may be 4 L of polyethylene glycol (GoLYTELY or Nu-LYTELY) or 45 ml of sodium phosphate (Fleets phospho-soda) mixed with one glass of water and followed by 3 glasses of water or juice. A second oral dose of this same preparation and an 8 oz glass of water at 6 a.m. on the day of the test.

On the morning of the test, baseline vital signs are taken and recorded.

• *During the Test*

Premedicate the patient with intravenous meperidine (Demerol), for analgesia and relaxation. This may be followed by intravenous diazepam (Valium), or intravenous midazolam (Versed). To prevent apnea, respiratory depression, or cardiac arrest, these medications must be given slowly over a period of 1 to 2 minutes. Naloxone (Narcan) is kept on hand to reverse the respiratory depressive effect of meperidine, but it is ineffective against diazepam.

Oxygen by nasal cannula increases the patient's oxygen reserves and helps prevent hypoxia.

Monitor the patient using the automated blood pressure, pulse oximeter, and ECG monitor. Monitor for an episode of vasovagal reflex that can occur with instrumentation. Atropine sulfate is kept on hand to overcome the effects of the sudden bradycardia.

Provide comfort and emotional support to help reduce anxiety and promote relaxation.

Assist with any collection of tissue specimens. The tissue is placed on filter paper and into a specimen container with fixative solution. Mark the label with the patient's name, date, source of tissue, and the procedure.

- *Posttest*

Monitor vital signs every 15 minutes or continue automated monitoring until the results are stable.

Check the rectal area for signs of blood.

Send the tissue specimen and requisition slip to the laboratory without delay.

As soon as the patient is more responsive, the intake of food and liquids can resume.

On discharge from an ambulatory care setting, the patient must be accompanied by a responsible person who will provide transportation home. The patient cannot drive a car for 8 to 12 hours because of the effects of medication.

☼ **COMPLICATION ALERT** ☼ Because hemorrhage and perforation can become apparent in the posttest period, the nurse assesses for signs of rectal bleeding, abdominal distension, persistent abdominal pain, or tenderness and malaise. If the condition is severe, the patient will develop hypotension and tachycardia.

COLPOSCOPY • ENDOSCOPY

N O R M A L   V A L U E S

No abnormalities of the vagina or cervix are noted.

Purpose of the Test

Colposcopy is performed to further evaluate an abnormal Papanicolaou's test (Pap smear), to monitor for precancerous abnormalities, or to evaluate a lesion of the vagina or cervix.

Procedure

The colposcope is inserted into the vagina. The endothelial and connective tissues are seen with magnification and illumination of the instrument. Cell samples are removed by endocervical curretage. A tissue biopsy may also be performed.

Findings

Atrophic cellular changes
Cervical erosion
Cervical intraepithelial neoplasia (CIN)
Condyloma
Invasive carcinoma
Papilloma

Interfering Factors

Vaginal creams
Menstruation

Nursing Implementation

• *Pretest*

To maximize visibility of the cervical tissue, schedule the procedure between days 8 and 12 of the menstrual cycle.
Instruct the patient to refrain from the application of any creams or vaginal medications because they obscure the view of the tissue.
To help reduce anxiety, provide specific information about the purpose of the test and the procedure.
Obtain written consent.

• *During the Test*

Place the patient in the lithotomy position with the legs supported in stirrups.
During the insertion of the colposcope, instruct the patient to breathe through the mouth to help relax the muscles.
Once the glass slides are prepared with cell scrapings, apply the fixative to prevent drying of the cells. If biopsy specimens are taken, place the tissue on hard brown paper or on a nonstick gauze (Telfa).

Each sample is placed in a separate specimen jar that contains fixative.

- Posttest

Label all specimens and write the source of the tissue on the requisition slip.

When a cervical biopsy is performed, instruct the patient to refrain from sexual intercourse and avoid the insertion of anything into the vagina until the lesion is healed.

COMPLEMENT, TOTAL (CH$_{50}$) • SERUM

NORMAL VALUES

75–160 U/ml *or* SI 75–160 kU/L

Purpose of the Test

Complement is a system of proteins that activate in conditions of inflammation and infection. This test is used to monitor systemic lupus erythematosus and its response to therapy. It is also used to diagnose complement deficiency and to detect autoimmune disease caused by the immune complex.

Procedure

A red-topped tube is used to collect 7 ml of venous blood.

Findings

Increase	*Decrease*
Chronic infection	Systemic lupus erythematosus
Rheumatoid arthritis	Multiple myeloma
Acute rheumatic fever	Acute glomerulonephritis
Ulcerative colitis	Hypogammaglobulinemia
Thyroiditis	Advanced cirrhosis of the liver

Interfering Factors

None

Nursing Implementation

No specific patient instruction or intervention is needed.

COMPLETE BLOOD COUNT (CBC) • BLOOD

N O R M A L   V A L U E S

WHITE BLOOD CELL COUNT (WBC)
$4.5–11 \times 10^3/\mu l$ or SI $4.5–11 \times 10^9/L$

RED BLOOD CELL COUNT (RBC)
Male: $4.6–6.2 \times 10^6/\mu L$ or SI $4.6–6.2 \times 10^{12}/L$
Female: $4.2–5.4 \times 10^6/\mu L$ or SI $4.2–5.4 \times 10^{12}/L$

HEMOGLOBIN
Male: 13.5–18 g/dl or SI 135–180 g/L
Female: 12–16 g/dl or SI 120–160 g/L

HEMATOCRIT
Male: 40–54% or SI 0.4–0.59 (volume fraction)
Female: 38–47% or SI 0.38–0.47 (volume fraction)

RED CELL INDICES
Mean corpuscular volume (MCV): 80–96 μm^3 or SI 80–96 fL
Mean corpuscular hemoglobin (MCH): 27–31 pg or SI 27–31 pg
Mean corpuscular hemoglobin concentration (MCHC): 32–36% or SI 0.32–0.36 (concentration fraction)
Red cell distribution width (RDW-CV): 13.1% (range: 11.6–14.6%) (Henry, 1996)

PLATELET COUNT
Adult: 150,000–450,000 cells/μL or SI $150–450 \times 10^9$

RETICULOCYTE COUNT
Adult: 25,000–75,000/μL or SI $25–75 \times 10^9/L$

Purpose of the Test

The CBC is used to assess the patient for anemia, infection, inflammation, polycythemia, hemolytic disease, the effects of ABO among different types of anemia, assess the severity of blood loss, and evaluate the bone marrow response to treatment of anemia.

Procedure

A purple-topped tube with EDTA anticoagulant is used to collect 7 ml of venous blood. As an alternative, two purple-tipped capillary tubes can be used to collect blood from a heelstick, earlobe, or finger puncture.

> ✓ QUALITY CONTROL
> For venipuncture, the tourniquet should be tied lightly for a brief time to prevent pooling of cells in the vein at the site of blood collection. To prevent hemolysis, the venipuncture technique must be smooth, with a blood flow that fills the vacuum tube readily. After the blood is collected, the tube is gently inverted 5 to 10 times to mix the anticoagulant and prevent clotting.

Findings

Increase	*Decrease*
White cell count	*White blood cells*
Infection	Aplastic anemia
Inflammation	Bone marrow depression
Leukemias	Pernicious anemia
Red cell count	Some infectious or parasitic
Polycythemia	diseases
Renal tumor	*Red blood cells*
Hemoconcentration	Hemorrhage
Hemoglobin	Hemodilution
Polycythemia	Anemia
Hemoconcentration	Aplastic anemia
Hematocrit	Bone marrow depression
Polycythemia	Hemolysis of erythrocytes
Hemoconcentration	*Hemoglobin*
Red cell indices	Hemorrhage
MCV: Pernicious anemia, vitamin B_{12} or folate deficiency	Anemia
	Hemolysis

Increase (cont.)

MCH: Hereditary spherocytosis

MCHC: Hereditary spherocytosis

RDW: Microcytic anemias

Platelets

Myeloproliferative diseases

Multiple myeloma

Iron deficiency anemia

Postsplenectomy response

Hodgkin's disease

Lymphomas

Renal disease

Infection or inflammation

Reticulocytes

Treatment for iron deficiency or pernicious anemia

Hemorrhage

Chronic blood loss

Hemolytic anemia

Decrease (cont.)

Hemodilution

Hematocrit

Hemorrhage

Anemia

Hemolysis

Hemodilution

Red cell indices

MCV: Iron deficiency anemia, chronic inflammation

MCH: Iron deficiency anemia

MCHC: Iron deficiency anemia

Platelets

Idiopathic thrombocytopenic purpura

Aplastic anemia

Anemias

Disseminated intravascular coagulation

Bone marrow depression

Systemic lupus erythematosus

Uremia

Liver disease

Reticulocytes

Aplastic anemia

Iron deficiency anemia

Anemia of chronic disease

Pernicious anemia

Endocrine or renal disease

Interfering Factors

Hemolysis

Coagulation of the specimen

Hemodilution

Frequent blood transfusion (reticulocyte count only)

Nursing Implementation

• *During the Test*

To prevent hemodilution from IV fluids, the blood is taken from the hand or arm that has no intravenous line.

• *Posttest*

Arrange for prompt transport of the specimen. If there is an anticipated delay, refrigerate the specimen.

COMPUTED TOMOGRAPHY	• RADIOLOGIC SCAN

Synonyms: CT scan, computerized axial tomography, CAT scan

NORMAL VALUES

No structural or anatomic abnormalities are noted.

Purpose of the Test

A CT scan uses a fan of x-ray beams to produce multiple images from many angles to form a 360-degree composite scan. CT provides precise visualization of the structure, size, shape, and density of soft tissue, bone, major blood vessels, and organs of the head and torso. It distinguishes between cyst, pseudocyst, benign and malignant tissue and is used in the staging of cancerous tumors. It can also be used to analyze the bone mineral content of the vertebrae in the assessment of osteoporosis. CT scans are part of the diagnostic work-up for severe headache, head trauma, hydrocephalus, suspicious space-occupying lesions, hemorrhage or edema, and suspected vascular lesions.

Procedure

With or without the use of an iodinated contrast medium, the patient moves through a scanner ring, and multiple x-ray beams pass through the tissue. As the x-ray photons fall on the scanner, images of the tissue are produced. Most organs can be scanned with or without contrast dye. Contrast dye is used usually to enhance visualization especially of the vasculature of the organ and is, therefore, indicated in certain clinical states. Depending on the speed of the scanner and the use or nonuse of contrast medium, the procedure requires 40 minutes to 2 hours to complete.

Findings

Tumor (benign, malignant)
Cyst
Stenosis

Thrombus
Embolus
Arteriosclerotic plaque
Necrotic sites
Calcification
Congenital malformation
Abscess
Calculus
Inflammation
Fluid collection
Bleeding or hemorrhage
Organ atrophy

Interfering Factors

Jewelry or metal in the x-ray field
Uncooperative patient behavior
Pregnancy
Failure to maintain a nothing-by-mouth status (if indicated)
Allergy to contrast material
Severe liver or kidney disease (with use of contrast medium)

Nursing Implementation

• *Pretest*

Ask the patient if there is any history of allergy to iodine or
shellfish or an allergic reaction to dye or contrast material
used in a previous x-ray study.

Explain the procedure to the patient and obtain written consent from the patient or person legally designated to make
health care decisions for the patient.

If contrast medium is to be used, instruct the patient to discontinue all food and fluids for 4 to 8 hours before the test.

Instruct the patient to remove all clothes, jewelry, and other
metal objects. A hospital gown is worn.

When no contrast material is used, reassure the patient that
the procedure is painless. With the use of contrast medium,
explain that the contrast agent is injected intravenously. The
patient may feel warmth at the injection site, a salty taste,
headache, or nausea as the agent is injected. These are temporary sensations that will disappear in a few minutes.

Provide appropriate orientation and reassurance so that fear of the unknown is diminished. Many patients feel some degree of apprehension as they enter the enclosed space of the machine.

Encourage the patient to relax during the scanning process by using techniques such as visual imagery, meditation, or prayer.

Sedatives are usually used for the infant or child less than 3 years old, particularly when the scan requires an extended period of immobility. Administer the prescribed sedative. The medication is usually chloral hydrate (by mouth or per rectum), or phenobarbital (intramuscularly).

• *During the Test*

Instruct the patient to remain motionless while in the scanner and to hold his or her breath when instructed to do so.

Keep an emesis basin in the nearby area in case the patient vomits after receiving the contrast medium.

• *Posttest*

If sedatives were administered, monitor the vital signs on a regular basis until the patient is responsive and awake.

No other special nursing measures are needed.

CORTISOL, PLASMA • PLASMA

N O R M A L   V A L U E S

ADULT
8 a.m.–10 a.m.: 5–23 µg/dl *or* SI 138–635 nmol/L
4 p.m.–6 p.m.: 3–13 µg/dl *or* SI 83–359 nmol/L

Purpose of the Test

The adrenal cortex produces a group of hormones called glucocorticoids. The primary glucocorticoid is cortisol. Secretion of cortisol is regulated by ACTH, which is secreted by the anterior pituitary gland. When secreted, most of the cortisol in the plasma binds with corticosteroid-binding globulin (CBG). The free cortisol is the biologically active form, whereas the bound hormone acts as a storehouse to replace the free cortisol.

Plasma cortisol levels are used to diagnose Cushing's syndrome, Cushing's disease, and primary and secondary adrenal insufficiency. Primary adrenal insufficiency is called Addison's disease. To distinguish between primary and secondary adrenal insufficiency, an *ACTH stimulation test (cosyntropin test, Cortrosyn stimulating test)* may be ordered.

Plasma cortisol levels are also used in the *dexamethosone (Decadron) suppression test*. This test assesses the hypothalamic-pituitary-adrenal axis. It distinguishes Cushing's disease (pituitary hypersecretion of ACTH) from adrenal tumors or ectopic secretion of ACTH. A variety of dexamethosone procedures are possible; however, they usually begin with a baseline plasma cortisol level, followed by the administration of dexamethasone. Then either a plasma cortisol level or urine sample for cortisol metabolites is obtained. No change will occur with adrenal tumors or ectopic ACTH production, since they are not dependent on ACTH stimulation.

Procedure

Venipuncture is performed to obtain 5 ml of blood in a green-topped tube. If instead of a plasma level, a serum level is desired, 5 ml of blood is collected in a red-topped tube. Varied methods are used to measure cortisol and include RIA, competitive protein-binding assay, fluorimetric assay, and high-performance liquid chromatography.

If an ACTH stimulation test is being done, after a baseline plasma cortisol level is obtained, cosyntropin (Cortrosyn) is given intravenously or intramuscularly. After 30 to 60 minutes, another plasma cortisol level is obtained. Normally, there is an increase in the plasma cortisol to $>18\mu g/dl$ (SI > 497 $\mu mol/L$). No change supports the diagnosis of primary adrenal disease.

Findings

Increase	*Decrease*
Stress	Addison's disease
Acute illness	Hypophysectomy
Surgery	Postpartum pituitary necrosis
Trauma	Pituitary destruction
Pregnancy	
Exogenous estrogen	
Anxiety	

Starvation
Anorexia nervosa
Alcoholism
Chronic renal failure

Interfering Factors

Noncompliance with dietary or activity restrictions, vary with the laboratory technique used:

With RIA
Androgens
Estrogens
Phenytoin
Hepatic dysfunction
Renal failure
With competitive protein-binding assay
Prednisolone
6-Alpha-methylprednisolone
With fluorimetric assays
Jaundice
Renal failure
Medications (niacin, quinacrine, quinidine, spironolactone)
With high-performance liquid chromatography
prednisone
prednisolone

Nursing Implementation

The nurse takes actions similar to those taken in plasma ACTH determinations (see p. 4).

• *Pretest*

Instruct the patient to limit physical activity for 12 hours before the test and to lie down for 30 minutes before the blood is drawn.

C-REACTIVE PROTEIN • SERUM

Synonym: CRP

N O R M A L   V A L U E S

<1 mg/dl *or* SI <10 mg/L

Purpose of the Test

C-reactive protein is used as a nonspecific indicator of infection or inflammation and also to monitor the response to antibiotic or anti-inflammatory medication. It is commonly used to help with the diagnosis of rheumatoid arthritis and rheumatic fever, particularly when the erythrocyte sedimentation rate (ESR) and other test results are inconclusive.

Procedure

A red-topped tube is used to collect 5 to 10 ml of venous blood.

> ✓ QUALITY CONTROL
> Venipuncture technique must be smooth, with a blood flow that fills the vacuum tube readily. If the blood has excessive turbulence because of flawed venipuncture technique, the hemolysis of the erythrocytes will alter the test results.

Findings

Increase

Rheumatoid arthritis
Rheumatic fever
Systemic lupus erythematosus
Bacterial sepsis
Tuberculosis
Pneumococcal pneumonia
Crohn's disease
Myocardial infarction

Interfering Factors

Oral contraceptives
Intrauterine device
Hemolysis

Nursing Implementation

• *Pretest*

Instruct the patient to fast from food for 4 to 8 hours before the test. Fluids are permitted. Fasting is required because for accurate results of serum lipid levels should be as low as possible.

• *Posttest*
No specific intervention is necessary.

CREATININE • SERUM

Synonyms: Plasma creatinine, Pcr

NORMAL VALUES

Adult male: 0.7–1.3 mg/dl *or* SI 62–115 µmol/L
Adult female: 0.6–1.1 mg/dl *or* SI 53–97 µmol/L
Adolescent: 0.5–1 mg/dl *or* SI 44–88 µmol/L
Child: 0.3–0.7 mg/dl *or* SI 27–62 µmol/L
Infant: 0.2–0.4 mg/dl *or* SI 18–35 µmol/L
Newborn: 0.3–1 mg/dl *or* SI 27–88 µmol/L

Purpose of the Test

A serum creatinine determination is the most common laboratory test used to evaluate renal function and to estimate the effectiveness of glomerular filtration. It is part of the routine blood chemistry screen or SMA (sequential multiple analyzer).

Procedure

A red-topped tube is used to collect 7 to 10 ml of venous blood. For infants and small children, a heelstick, earlobe, or finger prick is used to fill a capillary pipette.

✓ QUALITY CONTROL
Venipuncture technique must be smooth, with a blood flow that fills the vacuum tube readily. If the blood has excessive turbulence because of flawed technique, the hemolysis of the erythrocytes will alter the results.

Findings

Increase	*Decrease*
Acute or chronic renal failure	Advanced liver disease
Uremia or azotemia	Long-term corticosteroid therapy
Renal artery stenosis	Hyperthyroidism
Congestive heart failure	Muscular dystrophy
Shock	

Increase (cont.)	*Decrease (cont.)*
Dehydration	Paralysis
Urinary tract obstruction	Dermatomyositis
Acromegaly or gigantism	Polymyositis
Rhabdomyolysis	

Interfering Factors

Hemolysis
Warming of the specimen

Nursing Implementation

- *Pretest*

Instruct the patient to fast from food and fluids for 8 hours before the test when indicated by the laboratory protocol. In some methods of analysis, lipemia causes a false elevation. Recent meat ingestion can also cause a false elevation.

- *Posttest*

Arrange for prompt transport of the specimen to the laboratory.

✓ QUALITY CONTROL
In the laboratory, the serum must be separated from the cells promptly to avoid the formation of ammonia. The serum must be refrigerated until it is analyzed. Warming to greater than 30° C causes the creatinine level to falsely become elevated.

CREATININE CLEARANCE, 24-HOUR URINE	• URINE

Synonyms: Ccre, Ccr, urine creatinine

N O R M A L   V A L U E S

MEAN CREATININE CLEARANCE
Adult male: 1–2 g/day *or* SI 8.8–17.7 μmol/day
90–139 ml/minute/1.73 m² *or* SI 0.87–1.34 ml/second/m²
Adult female: 0.8–1.8 g/day *or* SI 7.1–15.9 μmol/day
80–125 ml/minute/1.73 m² *or* SI 0.77–1.2 ml/second/m²
Child: 70–140 ml/minute/1.73 m² *or* SI 1.17–2.33 ml/second/m²

Purpose of the Test

The urine creatinine clearance test is performed to help assess renal function and creatinine excretion. It is also used to monitor the progress of renal disease. The amount of urinary creatinine is increased significantly by muscle necrosis and muscle atrophy because of protein catabolism. It is decreased significantly in acute and advanced chronic renal failure because of the kidneys' inability to filter and excrete this waste product.

The urinary creatinine clearance test is usually accompanied by a serum creatinine test. The blood test may be performed at the midpoint in urinary collection or at the start and completion of the urine collection, depending on laboratory protocol.

Procedure

The test usually requires urine collection for 24 hours, but collection periods of 4 or 12 hours are sometimes prescribed.

Findings

Increase	*Decrease*
Muscular dystrophy	Glomerulonephritis
Polymyositis	Congestive heart failure
Paralysis	Acute tubular necrosis
Muscular inflammatory disease	Advanced pyelonephritis
	Shock
Hyperthyroidism	Polycystic kidney disease
Anemia	Renal malignancy
Leukemia	Dehydration
	Bilateral ureteral obstruction
	Nephrosclerosis

Interfering Factors

Excessive exercise in the test period
Failure to collect all the urine
Failure to time the test accurately
Warming of the urine specimen
High protein intake prior to the test

Nursing Implementation

• *Pretest*

Instruct the patient to avoid excessive intake of meat on the day before the test.

Instruct the patient to collect all urine for the 24-hour period of the test, storing the container in the refrigerator or on ice.

Encourage adequate hydration before and during the test, omitting coffee and tea during the test.

• *During the Test*

At 8 a.m., instruct the patient to void and discard the urine. The test begins at this time and all subsequent urine specimens are collected for 24 hours, including the 8 a.m. specimen of the next morning.

Advise the patient to avoid vigorous exercise during the test period.

Ensure that the patient's name and the time and date of the start and finish of the test are written on the label and requisition slip.

• *Posttest*

Arrange for prompt transportation of the refrigerated specimen to the laboratory.

CYSTOSCOPY • ENDOSCOPY

Synonyms: None

NORMAL VALUES

No anatomic or structural abnormalities are present.

Purpose of the Test

Cystoscopy provides direct visualization of the urinary bladder. When the urethra also is examined, the procedure is called *cystourethroscopy.*

Cystoscopy is used to investigate the cause of painless hematuria, particularly when cancer of the epithelial lining is suspected. It also is part of the investigation into the cause of urinary incontinence or retention. The examiner is able to visualize the location, extent, and exact nature of the problem. Following the diagnostic component, treatment may include dilation of stricture, cauterization of bleeding spots, removal of superficial tissue, implantation of radium seeds, and placement of a ureteral stent or catheter.

Procedure

Under local anesthesia, the cystoscope is inserted through the urethra into the urinary bladder. Once the bladder is filled with isotonic saline, all aspects of the bladder walls are examined with the lighted cystoscope. Biopsy samples for tissue examination and cell washings for cytologic analysis may be carried out. Urine samples may be collected from the bladder or from each ureter. The procedure takes 30 to 45 minutes.

Findings

Cancer of the bladder
Polyps
Diverticula of the bladder
Bladder fistula
Bladder stones
Bladder neck stricture
Congenital anomaly
Benign prostatic hypertrophy
Cancer of the prostate gland

Interfering Factors

Failure to maintain a nothing-by-mouth status
Acute infection of the bladder, urethra, or prostate gland

Nursing Implementation

• *Pretest*

Inform the patient about the procedure and obtain a written consent from the patient or person legally designated to make health care decisions for the patient.

When bowel emptying is part of the protocol, instruct the patient to administer an enema the night before or the morning of the test.

For general or spinal anesthesia preparation, instruct the patient to fast from food and fluid for 8 hours before the procedure. For local anesthesia, fasting from food is required, but clear liquids on the morning of the test are permitted.

Take baseline vital signs and record the results.

Preoperative sedatives or antispasmodics may be prescribed.

- *During the Test*

Provide reassurance to the patient who is awake during the procedure. The instillation of the local anesthetic into the urethra is mildly painful until the tissue becomes numb. When the bladder is filled with the irrigation solution, discomfort and the urge to void are normal sensations.

Assist with the collection of specimens. The biopsy tissue is placed in a sterile glass container with formalin preservative. For the cytologic study, 50 to 75 ml of bladder irrigation fluid is placed in a sterile jar with 50% alcohol as a preservative. Label specimen as bladder washings.

Assist with the collection of urine specimens and mark their source (bladder, right ureter, left ureter).

- *Posttest*

Take vital signs and record the results. For patients who have undergone general anesthesia, continue monitoring the vital signs every 15 to 30 minutes until the patient is stable.

Assess for pain or bladder spasms and medicate as needed.

Encourage extra oral fluids to promote adequate hydration and the voiding of urine.

Instruct the patient to void within 8 hours after the test.

Reassure the patient that it is normal to have a burning sensation on voiding and to see a small amount of blood or pink-tinged urine. These problems should disappear after the third voiding.

At home, warm tub baths can help alleviate the discomfort or pain of bladder spasms. Instruct the patient to avoid alcohol for 48 hours because of its irritant effect on the bladder mucosa.

To prevent infection, instruct the patient to take the prescribed antibiotic for 1 to 3 days.

Assess patient for complications: Bleeding, obstruction, and infection.

✪ **COMPLICATION ALERT** ✪ Since patients usually go home soon after the cystoscopy, the nurse needs to instruct the patient to report clinical manifestations of complications, including persistent hematuria, passage of blood clots, inability to void within 8 hours despite desire to void, flank or abdominal pain, chills, fever, and pyuria.

D

DARKFIELD EXAMINATION, SYPHILIS
● CELL SCRAPINGS

N O R M A L   V A L U E S

Negative

Purpose of the Test

The microscopic examination identifies the *Treponema pallidum* spirochete, the cause of a syphilis infection. This test gives an early diagnosis, before blood tests are reactive.

Procedure

Pipette Method. After the surface of the chancre is cleansed with a saline-moistened swab, a sterile pipette is used to aspirate cells and exudate from the base of the ulcer. The secretions are placed on a sterile glass slide.

Slide Method. After cleansing the surface of the chancre with a saline-moistened swab, a sterile glass slide is pressed directly on the ulcerated lesion.

✓ QUALITY CONTROL
Once the specimen is obtained, a coverslip is placed over the slide to prevent drying.

Findings

Positive. Syphilis infection

Interfering Factors

Contamination of the specimen
Drying of the specimen

Antibiotic therapy
Healed lesion

Nursing Implementation

• Pretest

Schedule this test before antibiotic therapy is started.
Instruct the patient to avoid placing lotions or creams on the lesion.

• During the Test

Wear gloves during the test and when handling the specimen slide. The lesion and secretions are contaminated.

• Posttest

Ensure immediate transport of the specimen to the laboratory. The darkfield examination must be performed within 15 minutes of collection, while the secretions are still moist.

Instruct the patient to abstain from sexual contact until the results are known and the infection is treated and cured.

When the test result is positive, instruct the patient to inform all sexual partners of the test results. Sexual contacts are advised to undergo testing.

Positive test results are reported to the state health department.

D-DIMER • PLASMA

NORMAL VALUES

Latex beads: <250 ng/ml *or* SI <250 µg/L
Enzyme-linked immunosorbent assay (ELISA): No D-dimer fragments are present

Purpose of the Test

The D-dimer test is used as a screening test for deep vein thrombosis. It helps determine whether a clot is present in the diagnosis of DIC, an acute myocardial infarction, and unstable angina. It is also used in the diagnosis of hypercoagulable conditions that cause recurrent thrombosis.

Procedure

A plastic syringe and a special plastic tube with sodium citrate and aprotinin additives are used to collect 4.5 ml of venous blood.

Findings

Increase

Thrombotic disease
DIC
Deep vein thrombosis
Sickle cell anemia crisis
Pulmonary embolism
Pregnancy (postpartum)
Arterial thromboembolism
Malignancy

Interfering Factors

None

Nursing Implementation

• *Posttest*

Arrange for immediate transport of the specimen to the laboratory. The patient is acutely ill and the test results are needed as quickly as possible.

DOPPLER ULTRASOUND • ULTRASOUND

Synonyms: Doppler flow studies, Doppler testing

N O R M A L   V A L U E S

ARTERIAL OR VENOUS EXAMINATION
Normal frequency and volume of audio signal
Normal waveform pattern
No evidence of vascular stenosis or obstruction

Purpose of the Test

Doppler ultrasound detects stenosis or occlusion in an artery or vein, assists with the diagnosis of peripheral artery or cerebrovascular disease, evaluates the results of arterial reconstruction or vascular bypass surgery, and assesses for possible trauma to an artery.

Doppler studies may be combined with radiographic imaging to detect and identify abnormalities of the arteries and veins. These are called duplex Doppler ultrasound (duplex scan, B-mode real-time imaging, duplex ultrasonography). B-mode imaging locates and provides images of the affected vessel, and the Doppler component identifies the disturbance of blood flow caused by atherosclerotic plaque or thrombus. The two methods are complementary; their combination provides information that is clearer than the data obtained from a single modality. Duplex Doppler ultrasound has been widely used to assess cranial neck vessels and now is also used to assess the abdominal aorta and the peripheral vascular system. The technique can detect an embolus, stenosis, a thrombus, an aneurysm, and venous insufficiency. It is used to verify the presence of deep vein thrombus, especially in the femoral and popliteal vein.

Procedure

The Doppler ultrasound probe transmits low-intensity sound waves that are directed at a specific blood vessel. The transmitted sound waves strike moving red blood cells and bounce back to the transducer-receiver within the probe. The received impulses are translated into an audible signal and a waveform recording on graph paper. Pressure readings are obtained from the waveforms.

Venous and Arterial Doppler Tests. Acoustic gel and the Doppler probe are placed on the skin at the desired vascular sites. Audible signals are heard and interpreted. Three to five waveforms are recorded at each vascular site. The specific vascular sites and sides of the body (right or left) are identified to avoid confusion and error. Venous sites of the lower extremities are the posterior tibial, greater saphenous, common femoral, superficial femoral, and popliteal veins. Venous sites of the upper extremities and neck are the brachial, axillary, subclavian, and jugular veins. Arterial pulse sites of the lower extremities are the common femoral, popliteal, dorsalis pedis, and posterior tibial pulses.

Arterial pulses in the upper extremities and neck are the brachial, radial, ulnar, and carotid pulses.

Findings

Arterial stenosis or occlusion
Venous thrombosis
Venous valvular incompetency

Interfering Factors

Nicotine
Alcohol
Caffeine
Anxiety
Uncooperative behavior

Nursing Implementation

- *Pretest*

Inform the patient about the test and obtain a written consent from the patient or the person legally designated to make health care decisions for the patient.

Instruct the patient to avoid nicotine, alcohol, caffeine, and other stimulants–depressants that will cause vasoconstriction.

Reduce the room lighting to promote relaxation.

Maintain a comfortable room temperature to prevent shivering and vasoconstriction.

Instruct the patient to remove all clothing and to wear a hospital gown.

For arterial tests, place the patient in the supine position. For venous tests of the lower extremities, position the patient in the supine position with two pillows under the legs to elevate them above the heart. The leg and hip are externally rotated and the knee is flexed.

- *During the Test*

Venous Doppler Examination

Apply acoustic gel to the skin at the ankle, calf, thigh, and groin.

At each test point, use the probe and the audio mode to listen to the blowing sound that is in rhythm with the respirations.

Record three to five venous waveforms at each site, labeling each recording with the correct anatomic location.

Arterial Doppler Examination

Locate the pulse points on the upper or lower extremities and apply acoustic gel.

At each pulse point, apply the probe and the audio mode to listen to the blowing sounds.

Record three to five arterial waveforms at each site, labeling
each recording with the correct anatomic location.

• *Posttest*

Remove the acoustic gel from the skin.

E

ECHOCARDIOGRAM • SONOGRAM

Synonyms: ECHO, heart sonogram, transthoracic echocardiogram

N O R M A L   V A L U E S

No anatomic or functional abnormalities

Purpose of the Test

An echocardiogram is a noninvasive test that uses ultrasound techniques to detect enlargement of the cardiac chambers or variations in chamber size during the cardiac cycle. An echocardiogram is performed for a variety of diagnostic reasons, such as to evaluate abnormal heart sounds; evaluate heart size, chamber size, and valvular function; and detect tumors, pericardial effusion, and wall motion abnormalities.

For a better view of the posterior atrium and aorta, a *transesophageal echocardiography* (TEE) may be done. Transesophageal echocardiography is also indicated when a transthoracic approach is inadequate, such as when the patient is obese or has chest wall structure abnormalities. Indications for transesophageal echocardiography include diagnosis of (1) a thoracic aortic pathologic condition, including suspected aneurysms; (2) mitral valve disease or assessment of a prosthetic valve; (3) suspected endocarditis; (4) congenital heart disease, for example, atrial septal defect; (5) left atrial intracardiac thrombi; and (6) cardiac tumors.

Because of the significant number of false positive cardiac stress test results, especially in middle age women, *exercise stress echocardiography* is being done. A stress ECHO is done in combination with exercise stress testing or with dobutamine stress testing. Exercise or dobutamine is used to raise the pulse to over 85% of the maximum heart rate (220 minus the person's age). If dobutamine does not raise heart rate to the desired rate, atropine IV is given. Atropine should *not* be given if the patient has had a recent myocardial infarction or is in atrial fibrillation. An ECHO is done before the stress testing, then at each 3-minute stage. Nursing care is similar as for stress testing.

Procedure

An echocardiogram may be carried out at the bedside, in a special laboratory, in a clinic, or in a doctor's office. A transducer is placed over the third and fourth intercostal spaces to the left of the sternum. The transducer emits ultrasonic beams of high-frequency sound waves that are inaudible to the human ear. The transducer then picks up the echos created by the deflection of the beams from the various heart structures. This creates a picture on the oscilloscope. The picture is created because the echo varies in intensity based on the differing densities of the structures.

Transesophageal echocardiography is similar to transthoracic echocardiography except that the ultrasound probe is fitted into the end of a flexible gastroscopy tube and advanced down the esophagus behind the heart.

Findings

Abnormal heart valves
Aneurysm
Cardiomyopathy
Congenital heart disorders
Congestive heart failure
Idiopathic hypertrophic subaortic stenosis
Mural thrombi
Myocardial infarction
Pericardial effusion
Restrictive pericarditis
Tumor of the heart

Interfering Factors

Chest wall abnormalities
Excessive movement
Improper placement of transducer

For a TEE

History of irradiation of mediastinum
Esophageal dysphagia
Structural abnormalities

Nursing Implementation

Transthoracic ECHO

- *Pretest*

Instruct the patient that the test is noninvasive. The patient
is awake during the test and usually in a recumbent position.

Inform the patient that an electromechanical transducer will
be positioned on the chest. The patient will sense only the
conduction jelly and the movement of the transducer. No
pain or risk is involved.

- *During the Test*

The patient may be asked to breathe slowly or hold the breath.

- *Posttest*

Evaluate the patient's response to the procedure.
Cleanse the chest of conduction gel.

Transesophageal ECHO

- *Pretest*

Ask patient is they have any history of or disorder of the esophagus, stomach, vocal cords, or throat. Ask if the patient has
any symptoms of infection of the mouth or throat. Report if
positive history is given.

Question patient about the presence of dentures, bridges, or
dental plates. Ask if there is any arthritis of the neck, respiratory problems, or if the patient is on anticoagulant therapy.
Document any medication allergies.

Ensure that a signed informed consent form has been obtained.

Maintain the patient on a nothing-by-mouth status for 6 to
8 hours.

Describe the procedure to the patient, especially the need for a mouthguard, positioning, and the need to swallow when asked.

If the patient has prosthetic heart valves, prophylactic antibiotics may be prescribed.

Administer antianxiety medication as prescribed.

• *During the Test*

Administer medication to decrease secretions as ordered.

A topical anesthetic is sprayed into the throat.

Instruct the patient to gargle with viscous lidocaine and then to swallow it. Warn the patient that it will make the tongue and throat feel "swollen."

A mouthguard is placed to prevent the patient from biting down on the endoscope or the physician's fingers.

The patient is positioned on the left side in the chin-chest position. The head may be supported with a small pillow.

The probe is lubricated with lidocaine jelly and slowly inserted as the patient swallows.

Monitor the patient for a vasovagal response from the medication given to dry up secretions.

Check the patient for gagging.

Observe the oximeter for oxygen saturation readings.

Observe for complications related to placement of the probe in the esophagus: esophageal bleeding, transient dysrhythmias, transient hypoxia, and vasovagal response.

❂ **COMPLICATION ALERT** ❂ Because of the possibility of hypoxia during a TEE, the nurse should place the patient on a pulse oximetry. Ensure the alarm limits are set.

• *Posttest*

Assess the patient for return of the gag reflex before resuming oral intake. Hot liquids are not given for at least 2 hours.

Give lozenges for relief of throat discomfort.

If done as an outpatient procedure, patient must be accompanied by another when discharged. Instruct patient not to drive for 6 to 12 hours after procedure.

ELECTROCARDIOGRAM

Synonyms: ECG, EKG, 12- or 18-lead ECG or EKG

NORMAL VALUES

Normal rate and rhythm. No abnormalities noted.

Purpose of the Test

The ECG is an invaluable tool in the assessment of the heart. It records the heart's electric activity. A 12-lead ECG presents a graphic recording of twelve electric planes of the heart. By manipulating the skin electrodes, twelve various views of the heart's electric activity are seen. If a right ventricular infarction is suspected, a 18-lead ECG is done. With the 18-lead ECG, six additional leads are recorded on the right chest, which mirror the placement of the 12-lead chest leads.

The purpose of the 12- and 18-lead ECG is to diagnose myocardial infarction, injury, and ischemia. It also assists in identifying hypertrophy, axis deviations, and electrolyte abnormalities and distinguishes between ventricular and supraventricular tachycardias. Left versus right hypertrophy can be distinguished by comparing the morphologic characteristics of the QRS complex in leads V_5 and V_6, by determining axis deviation, and by the P wave.

Holter Monitoring. Also called *ambulatory monitoring,* it permits the recording of cardiac electric activity over time (usually 24 hours) on a cassette tape recorder. It allows the patient to perform normal daily activities so that cardiac responses to these activities can be determined.

The primary purpose of Holter monitoring is dysrhythmia detection. These procedures are helpful in identifying conduction defects and responses to therapeutic measures.

Procedure

For a 12- and 18-lead ECG, the technician, the physician, or the nurse places the patient in a supine position. Conduction jelly is placed on the electrodes, and the electrodes are applied. The electrocardiograph's electrode wires are marked and color-coded. The limb lead electrodes are placed on the arms and legs.

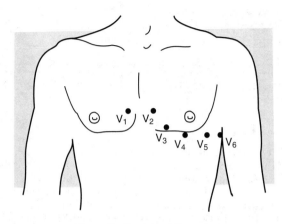

Figure 3. Chest Lead Placement.

It is essential that the chest leads be positioned correctly for accurate interpretation (see Fig. 3).

The chest leads for the 12-lead ECG are applied as follows:

V_1: Fourth intercostal space at the right sternal border
V_2: Fourth intercostal space at the left sternal border
V_3: Midway between V_2 and V_4
V_4: Fifth intercostal space at the left midclavicular line
V_5: Fifth intercostal space at the anterior axillary line
V_6: Fifth intercostal space at the midaxillary line

Electrocardiographs vary. Older machines record one lead at a time. Newer machines simultaneously record the twelve leads and automatically mark the leads.

With Holter monitoring, electrodes are applied to the patient's chest (placement varies with desired leads) and attached to a battery-operated tape recorder. Most recorders permit simultaneous recording of two channels (frequently lead II and V_5 are chosen). Recorders are equipped with an event marker, which alerts the scanning technician that the patient experienced some symptom. A diary is kept by the patient, who records daily activities and the times they were performed, when and what medications were taken, and the presence and time symptoms occurred. The recordings are analyzed at 60 to 120 times real time by a microcomputer program. Any abnormalities are then recorded on the usual electrocardiograph paper.

Findings

Axis deviations (right or left)
Conduction disturbances
Dysrhythmias
Hypertrophy of the ventricles
Electrolyte imbalances
Pericarditis
Pulmonary infarctions
Therapeutic drug effects or toxicity, or both
As a myocardial infarction evolves, a sequence of electrocardiographic changes occurs. First, the ST segment changes. Elevation of an ST segment indicates myocardial injury. ST depression occurs as a reciprocal change in the ventricular wall opposite the infarction. The ST segment will return to normal within days or weeks after the infarction. Within hours or days of the infarction, the T wave inverts. It reflects ischemic changes in the heart. The T wave will revert back to normal within weeks or months of the infarction. Lastly, an abnormal Q wave appears in the leads directly over the transmural myocardial infarction. An abnormal Q wave is the presence of a Q wave in a lead in which a Q wave is not normally seen or one that is wider than 0.04 seconds or a third of the height of the QRS complex. A nonQ-wave infarction occurs when there is a subendocardial infarction. A Q wave indicates myocardial necrosis and may remain for years after the infarction.

Table 1 summarizes which leads reflect which walls of the left

TABLE 1. Electrocardiographic Changes with Acute Myocardial Infarction

	Lead Changes	Reciprocal Changes
Inferior wall	II, III, aVF	I, aVL
Lateral wall	I, aVL, V$_5$, V$_6$	V$_1$, V$_2$, V$_3$
Anterior wall	V$_2$, V$_3$, V$_4$	II, III, aVF
Anteroseptal	V$_1$, V$_2$, V$_3$, V$_4$	II, III, aVF
Posterior wall		V$_1$, V$_2$, V$_3$, V$_4$

ventricle. Note that since no leads are usually placed over the posterior wall of the heart, posterior infarctions are diagnosed by reciprocal changes.

Right ventricular infarctions are assessed by performing a right-sided ECG, which indicates ST elevations in V_{4R} and V_{5R}.

✓ QUALITY CONTROL

If a right ventricular infarction is suspected, the right-sided ECG must be done within 10 hours of the infarction (occurrence of chest pain). The ST segment changes return to normal very quickly after the infarction.

Interfering Factors

Patient movement, poor grounding, and poor skin contact can interfere with a clear recording of the ECG.

Nursing Implementation for a 12- and 18-Lead Electrocardiogram

• *Pretest*

Explain to the patient the purpose and procedure for the ECG. No risk is involved.

No pretest restrictions are required.

Since electrodes are applied to the four extremities and the chest, clothing should permit easy access. If the patient's chest is excessively hairy, the sites may need to be shaved.

• *During the Test*

Establish a relaxed environment.

Place the patient in a supine position.

Conduction jelly is placed on the electrodes and the electrodes are applied.

The recording is made.

• *Posttest*

Remove the conduction jelly.

Help the patient to a comfortable position.

Nursing Implementation for Holter Monitoring

• *Pretest*

Inform the patient as to the purpose of the Holter monitor.

Instruct patient on use of the event marker and to maintain a diary of activities and symptoms.

Apply the electrodes as indicated usually for lead II and V_5.
  Shave the site if the chest is hairy.

• *During the Test*

Check monitor's indicator light to determine if battery is functioning.

• *Posttest*

Remove electrodes and cleanse site of jelly.
Observe skin for signs of irritation.

ELECTROENCEPHALOGRAPHY • ELECTROPHYSIOLOGY

Synonyms: Electroencephalogram, EEG

N O R M A L   V A L U E S

Normal patterns of electric brain activity are seen.

Purpose of the Test

Electroencephalography records the spontaneous brain activity that originates from the cortical pyramidal cells on the surface of the brain. The electric activity, called action potential, comes from the depolarization of nerve cell membranes. The fluctuations of electric activity from the larger cortical areas of the brain are detected on the electroencephalogram (EEG).

Using the older electroencephalographic methodology, the fluctuations in electric activity are recorded on a moving paper by a series of pens. In several of the newer methodologies, the data are computerized and displayed on a monitor and can be videotaped.

The major applications of the EEG are in the diagnosis of epilepsy, the determination of the type of epilepsy, the diagnosis of metabolic encephalopathy, and in identifying brain injury. EEG is also used in protocols for defining brain death.

Procedure

In adults, twenty-one recording needle electrodes are applied to the scalp in particular groupings, using electric paste to promote conduction. The electrode wires are connected to the electroencephalograph recorder. In neonates, fewer electrodes are used because of the smaller head size. The electroencephalography procedure may take several hours. The patient may be asked to blink or swallow during the procedure. Some patients' EEGs are done during sleep or may be done after the patients are deprived of sleep.

For the neonate, the test is usually performed in the isolette in the neonatal intensive care unit.

Findings

Epilepsy (grand mal, focal, temporal lobe, myoclonal, petit mal)
Cerebral infarct
Intracranial hemorrhage
Brain death
Ischemic encephalopathy
Brain tumor

Interfering Factors

Caffeine
Movements of the hands, body, or tongue
Muscle contractions
Drug intoxication (heroin, cocaine, marijuana, crack, lysergic acid diethylamide [LSD])
Hypoglycemia
Particular medications (narcotics, sedatives, tranquilizers, monoamine oxidase inhibitors, anticonvulsants, antihistamines)
Soiling of scalp (hair spray, oils, etc.)

Nursing Implementation

• *Pretest*

Instruct the patient to avoid caffeine before the test because stimulants alter the electroencephalographic activity. A light meal and fluid intake are encouraged because a low blood glucose level can also alter the electroencephalographic results.

Instruct the patient to wash his or her hair thoroughly before the test.

If a sleep-deprived EEG is performed to evaluate sleep disorder or seizures that occur during sleep, advise the patient not to sleep on the night before the test. At the time of the test, a sedative may be given to promote sleep. If this form of EEG is used, advise the patient to have a responsible person available to drive him or her home after the test is completed.

Since anticonvulsants and other sedative medications alter the electric activity of the brain, these medications may be withheld for 24 to 48 hours before the test begins, as determined by the physician. If the medications cannot be withheld because of the seriousness of the patient's seizure disorder, all medications taken in the 24- to 48-hour pretest period are documented on the requisition slip.

• During the Test

Help the patient to relax in the reclining chair or bed.

Inform the patient that a prickly sensation or temporary pain is felt as the electrodes are attached to the scalp. Reassure the patient that the electrodes and wires will not cause a shock or harm the patient.

Instruct the patient not to move the head or body and not to talk during the test. These muscle movements alter the electroencephalographic readings. For the neonate, place the head in a midline alignment.

Reassure the patient that the nurse is nearby, in full visibility of the patient during the procedure. If a seizure occurs, the nurse is prepared to provide care during the episode.

• Posttest

Observe the patient for seizure activity.

Remove the electrodes. The electrode paste is cleaned from the hair and scalp by using acetone and cotton balls. Acetone is not used in the isolette because of the limited circulation of air.

Anticonvulsant medications that were withheld for the test are not automatically restarted at the same dosage. Previous orders are reviewed by the physician and a new set of orders are written.

ELECTROLYTES, 24-HOUR URINE   • URINE

Synonyms: Sodium, chloride, potassium

N O R M A L   V A L U E S

SODIUM
Adult: 40–220 mEq/24 hours *or* SI 40–220 μmol/24 hours
Child (6–10 years)
Male: 41–115 mEq/24 hours *or* SI 41–115 μmol/24 hours
Female: 20–69 mEq/24 hours *or* SI 20–69 μmol/24 hours
Child (10–14 years)
Male: 63–117 mEq/24 hours *or* SI 63–117 μmol/24 hours
Female: 48–168 mEq/24 hours *or* SI 48–168 μmol/24 hours

CHLORIDE
Adult: 110–250 mEq/24 hours *or* SI 110–250 μmol/24 hours
Adult (>60 years): 95–195 mEq/24 hours *or* SI 95–195 μmol/24 hours
Child (<6 years): 15–40 mEq/24 hours *or* SI 15–40 μmol/24 hours
Child (6–10 years)
Male: 36–110 mEq/24 hours *or* SI 36–110 μmol/24 hours
Female: 18–74 mEq/24 hours *or* SI 18–74 μmol/24 hours
Child (10–14 years)
Male: 64–176 mEq/24 hours *or* SI 64–176 μmol/24 hours
Female: 36–173 mEq/24 hours *or* SI 36–173 μmol/24 hours
Infant: 2–10 mEq/24 hours *or* SI 2–10 μmol/24 hours

POTASSIUM
Adult: 25–125 mEq/24 hours *or* SI 25–125 μmol/24 hours
Child (6–10 years)
Male:17–54 mEq/24 hours *or* SI 17–54 μmol/24 hours
Female: 8–37 mEq/24 hours *or* SI 8–37 μmol/24 hours
Child (10–14 years)
Male: 22–57 mEq/24 hours *or* SI 22–57 μmol/24 hours
Female: 18–58 mEq/24 hours *or* SI 18–58 μmol/24 hours
Infant: 4.1–5.3 mEq/24 hours *or* SI 4.1–5.3 μmol/24 hours

Purpose of the Test

Urine electrolytes are used to help monitor renal function, fluid
and electrolyte balance, and acid-base balance.

Procedure

A 24-hour urine specimen is collected in a large, clean urine collection container. Alternative methods include a 12-hour urine collection or a single random urine sample for electrolyte testing. If a 24-hour urine test for protein or creatinine clearance is also ordered, these tests can be performed simultaneously with the urine electrolyte test, using the same specimen.

Findings

Increase in Sodium and Chloride

Increased sodium chloride intake
Adrenal failure
Addison's disease
Nephritis (salt-wasting)
Renal tubular acidosis
Syndrome of inappropriate antidiuretic hormone
Alkalosis
Diuretic therapy
Acute or chronic renal failure

Increase in Potassium

Increased potassium intake
Cushing's syndrome
Aldosterone
Renal tubular disease
Metabolic acidosis
Adrenocorticotropic hormone or cortisone treatment
Salicylate poisoning

Decrease in Sodium and Chloride

Decreased sodium chloride intake
Cushing's syndrome
Cirrhosis (with ascites)
Congestive heart failure
Nephrotic syndrome
Prerenal azotemia
Vomiting
Diarrhea
Intestinal fistula
Severe burns
Excessive sweating
Metabolic acidosis

Decrease in Potassium

Addison's disease
Acute glomerulonephritis
Pyelonephritis
Nephrosclerosis
Malabsorption syndrome
Metabolic alkalosis

Interfering Factors

Blood in the urine
Warming of the specimen

Nursing Implementation

• *Pretest*

Obtain a urine collection container from the laboratory for the collection of all urine in the 24-hour test period.

• *During the Test*

Instruct the patient to void at 8 a.m. and discard the specimen. The test begins immediately thereafter, and all urine is collected for the next 24 hours, including the 8 a.m. specimen of the next morning.

Keep the urine in the refrigerator or on ice throughout the collection period.

Ensure that the patient's name, the date, and the time of the start and finish of the test are written on the label and the requisition slip.

• *Posttest*

Arrange for prompt transport of the chilled specimen to the laboratory.

ELECTROMYOGRAPHY— NERVE CONDUCTION STUDIES	• ELECTROPHYSIOLOGY

Synonyms: EMG, NCS, electrodiagnostic studies

NORMAL VALUES

The muscle shows minimal activity at rest. Nerve conduction time is within normal limits.

Purpose of the Test

When a patient complains of muscle weakness, muscle spasms, or paralysis, the cause may be disease of the muscle or nervous system or a problem with neuromuscular transmission at the junction between the nerves and the muscle fibers. Electromyography (EMG) and nerve conduction studies are two diagnostic tests that help identify the physiologic location of the problem.

These tests help distinguish among the causes of weakness and paralysis, differentiating nerve involvement from a muscle disorder. The tests are also used to identify the particular nerve or muscle group that is involved, localize the site of the abnormality, evaluate the severity, and distinguish sensorimotor nerve disorder from pure motor disorder.

Electromyography. This procedure records the electric potential of various muscles in a resting state and during voluntary contraction of the muscles. The linear recordings are comparable to electrocardiographic recordings. The normal tracings of muscle potential demonstrate characteristic patterns at rest and during a strong voluntary muscle contraction. The recordings of "motor unit potentials" are examined for amplitude, duration, form, and abundance. Characteristic abnormal patterns are seen when the problem is neurologic in origin, such as denervation, or muscular, such as muscle inflammation.

Nerve Conduction Studies. These studies measure motor conduction velocity and sensory conduction. Motor conduction velocity is the timed measurement of conduction along a nerve between two points, as measured by the stimulating and recording electrodes that are applied on the nerve's pathway. Sensory conduction measures the voltage or strength of the nerve stimulus in sensory nerve endings by recording electrodes applied to a distal area of tissue.

Procedure

Needle electrodes are inserted into muscles and connected to stimulator and recorder devices. As the electric stimulus is initiated, the results appear on an oscilloscope or videoscreen or are photographed. Linear tracings of the electromyography are made by the electromyograph equipment.

The electrodiagnostic tests are somewhat painful and provoke some anxiety. The discomfort is sharp, but it is brief in duration. The pain is caused by the needle insertions and the electric stimuli. Sedation is not recommended because it interferes with voluntary muscle activity.

For infants and children, the process of testing is similar to that of adults, with some modifications because of the smaller body size.

Findings

Amyotrophic lateral sclerosis
Muscular dystrophy
Myasthenia gravis
Poliomyelitis
Inflammatory myositis
Myopathy (endocrine, metabolic, toxic, congenital)
Hypothyroidism
Botulism
Herniated lumbar disc
Guillain-Barré syndrome
Carpal tunnel syndrome
Brachial plexus injury
Lumbosacral plexus injury
Nerve trauma
Glycogen storage disease

Interfering Factors

Smoking
Caffeine
Acute anxiety

Nursing Implementation

- *Pretest*

Obtain written consent from the patient or person legally responsible for the patient's health care decisions.

Instruct the patient to refrain from smoking for 24 hours before the test and to avoid caffeine (coffee, tea, cola) for 2 to 3 hours before the test.

Inform the patient that the insertion of the needles can be painful and that the small shocks are also painful. Reassure the patient that these sensations are brief and can be tolerated.

If possible, encourage the parent to comfort the child during the procedure.

- *During the Test*

Cleanse the skin with antiseptic before inserting the electrodes.

As the electrodes are inserted, again reassure the patient, to help reduce anxiety.

For grounding, place a metal plate under the patient's body.

At appropriate intervals during EMG, ask the patient to perform various voluntary muscle contractions.

- *Posttest*

To avoid additional pain, remove the needle electrodes gently and slowly.

If pain persists at the puncture sites, instruct the patient to apply warm compresses.

ELECTROPHYSIOLOGIC STUDIES • RADIOLOGY

Synonym: EPS

NORMAL VALUES

Normal cardiac rhythm
Normal conduction, refractory, and interval times

Purpose of the Test

Electrophysiologic studies are performed to diagnose dysrhythmias, identify causes of ectopy, and determine a person's risk for lethal ventricular dysrhythmias. They are used to determine appropriate therapy in patients who have not obtained the desired effect from usual therapies and in whom noninvasive evaluation techniques have not provided the information necessary to determine which therapy or combination of therapies will be effective.

Procedure

Several procedures are included in the category of electrophysiologic studies. The patient may have one or all of the studies performed based on the clinical state. During the test, three or four multipolar pacing catheters are inserted percutaneously. One is positioned high in the atrium, one in the low-septal right atrium, one in the coronary sinus, and one in the right ventricle. Conduction intervals are measured to locate conduction delays by *programmed electrical stimulation* (PES). Atrial pacing is carried out to assess sinoatrial node response, AV node response, and bundle of His and Purkinje conduction. If indicated, *atrial extrastimulus testing* (AEST) is performed. With this test, a premature atrial stimulus is initiated to assess atrial and AV node response. Atrial flutter or atrial fibrillation may be initiated. The focus or reentry pathway may then be identified. In some patients, *His bundle electrographic studies* are performed to evaluate His bundle conduction.

Ventricular extrastimulus testing (VEST) is performed to assess ventricular dysrhythmias. Ventricular tachycardia (VT) may be induced. If a right ventricular stimulus does not induce VT, a left-sided stimulation may be carried out. This requires the insertion of a multipolar pacing catheter through an artery. When VT is induced, its response to overdrive pacing or drugs, or both, can be evaluated. If the patient has recurrent VT, *ventricular endocardial mapping* may be performed to localize the origin of the dysrhythmia. If ventricular mapping is performed, VT is induced and the ectopic focus is delineated by multiple intracardiac tracings.

If the electrophysiologic studies involve evaluation of drug responses, the test must be repeated because only one drug or combination of drugs can be assessed at a time. If this is necessary, subclavian catheters are left in place between testings.

Findings

Electrophysiologic studies may identify dysrhythmias, conduction abnormalities, and appropriate treatment for these disturbances.

Interfering Factors

See section on cardiac catheterization (pp. 67–71).

Nursing Implementation

The nursing actions are similar to those for cardiac catheterization with the following additions.

- *Pretest*

Reassure the patient that if dysrhythmias or blocks occur, resources are available to control and treat them.

Warn the patient that a "fluttering" sensation in the chest or hiccups may occur.

Antiarrhythmic drugs are usually discontinued for four half-lives (or four doses) before the test. In patients with potentially lethal dysrhythmias, cardiac monitoring is required.

The patient receives nothing by mouth for 6 hours prior to the procedure.

Premedication usually consists of diazepam (Valium), since it has no significant electrophysiologic effect. Avoid any medications with possible cardiac effect.

- *During the Test*

Actions are similar to those in cardiac catheterization except that only small doses of lidocaine are used as a local anesthetic to prevent systemic effects.

If ventricular tachycardia is induced, the nurse speaks with the patient to assess cerebral perfusion.

- *Posttest*

Assess site of catheter placement. If further studies are to be carried out, a catheter may have been left in place.

Check distal pulses if left-sided catheterization was performed.

Bed rest is maintained. For a right-sided study, bed rest is maintained for 2 hours; for a left-sided study, bed rest is maintained for 6 to 12 hours.

Encourage the patient to turn from side to side.

Avoid hip flexion if a femoral insertion was performed.

Evaluate the dressings for bleeding and infection. They should be kept dry and intact.

Anticoagulant therapy may be ordered if prolonged catheterization was required or if left ventricular stimulation or mapping was performed.

Patient and family teaching will depend on the findings of the studies and the indicated therapy.

Observe patient for complications, which are similar to a cardiac catheterization.

ENDOMYOCARDIAL BIOPSY • PATHOLOGY

N O R M A L   V A L U E S

Normal cardiac tissue

Purpose of the Test

Endomyocardial biopsy is an invasive procedure requiring cardiac catheterization. It permits sampling of right or left ventricular tissue. An endomyocardial biopsy is usually performed to determine if a transplanted heart is being rejected. Other purposes for the biopsy are to diagnose myocarditis or doxorubicin (Adriamycin) cardiomyopathy and to determine the cause of restrictive heart disease.

Procedure

The procedure involves a cardiac catheterization (see pp. 67–71). A catheter with a jaw-like tip is inserted under fluoroscopy, and several small tissue samples are obtained. A right or left ventricular sample may be taken. For patients at high risk, such as those with a history of left ventricular thrombus or infarction, a right ventricular biopsy may be preferred.

Findings

Doxorubicin-induced cardiomyopathy
Cardiac amyloidosis
Cardiac fibrosis (especially radiation injury)
Chagas' cardiomyopathy
Myocarditis
Rejection of transplanted heart
Scleroderma
Toxoplasmosis
Tumor infiltrates
Vasculitis

Interfering Factors

Bleeding disorders
Severe thrombocytopenia
Systemic anticoagulation
Uncooperative patient

Nursing Implementation

See discussion of cardiac catheterization (pp. 69–71).

✪ COMPLICATION ALERT ✪ Although complications of endomyocardial biopsy are rare, they include accidental biopsy of papillary muscle or chordae tendineae, cardiac perforation, and hemopericardium. The nurse assesses cardiac tamponade, decreased cardiac output, and new onset of a mitral or tricuspid murmur. Other complications can occur but are related to the catheterization rather than the biopsy itself.

ENDOSCOPIC RETROGRADE CHOLANGIOPANCREATOGRAPHY	• ENDOSCOPY

Synonym: ERCP

N O R M A L   V A L U E S

The ductal systems of the gallbladder, liver, and pancreas are patent, with no evidence of obstruction from stone, stricture, or tumor.

Purpose of the Test

ERCP is used to investigate the cause of obstructive jaundice and/or persistent abdominal pain associated with biliary or pancreatic disorder.

Procedure

A fiberoptic endoscope is passed through the mouth, esophagus, stomach, and into the duodenum. A small canula is inserted into the ampulla of Vater and then into the common duct and pancreatic duct. In each main duct, radiopaque dye is instilled and x-rays taken to demonstrate the filling of that duct. Pancreatic secretions may be collected for cytologic examination.

> ✓ QUALITY CONTROL
> Before the examination starts, the nurse tests all equipment for correct mechanical function and proper illumination. The imaging systems must also be fully operational. Backup equipment is kept available to prevent malfunction.

Findings

Biliary stone
Sclerosing cholangitis
Fibrosis or stricture
Cholangiocarcinoma
Metastatic cancer
Chronic pancreatitis
Cancer of the head of the pancreas
Fistula
Abscess

Interfering Factors

Uncooperative behavior
Severe, acute pancreatitis
Acute biliary obstruction
Acute myocardial infarction
Esophageal or gastric outlet obstruction
Hepatitis B infection

Nursing Implementation

- *Pretest*

Provide teaching so that the patient can cooperate during the examination. Intravenous medication will be given to provide relaxation and analgesia. An informed consent must be signed by the patient or the person legally responsible for the patient's health care decisions.

Take and record the patient's baseline vital signs.

Question the patient regarding any history of allergy to iodine, seafood, or previous reaction to dye used in an x-ray study.

Inform the patient to discontinue all foods and fluids for 12 hours before the test.

One hour before the start of the procedure, an intravenous infusion is started in the arm or hand.

When cholangitis or infection are suspected, systemic antibiotics are started and continued into the postprocedure period.

Intravenous diazepam (Valium), meperidine (Demerol), and atropine are used to provide relaxation, analgesia, and reduced motility of the intestinal tract. Alternatively, a bolus dose of midazolam (Versed) exerts a powerful, rapid enhancement of the narcotic. It also provides sedation and amnesia.

Begin to monitor the vital signs and respiratory status using the automated blood pressure, pulse oximetry, and cardiac monitor equipment.

Prior to the insertion of the endoscope, the patient's mouth and throat are anesthetized with a topical spray. An oral brace is inserted into the mouth to keep it open; a suction catheter is inserted to remove saliva.

• During the Test

Record the frequent assessments of the patient's cardiovascular and respiratory status. Oxygen is administered by nasal canula. Hypoxemia and bradycardia can occur.

✓ QUALITY CONTROL

To prevent respiratory depression or cardiac arrest, naloxone (Narcan) is kept on hand to reverse the respiratory depressive effect of meperidine. Atropine is immediately available in the event of an episode of bradycardia.

✓ QUALITY CONTROL

On completion of the procedure, the laparoscope must be disassembled, thoroughly cleaned, and disinfected. Since the instrument is reused, these measures prevent transmission of infection.

• Posttest

Monitor the cardiovascular and respiratory status at 15-minute intervals until the patient is stable.

The patient remains NPO until the gag reflex and swallowing ability return. Then, clear fluids are started and a light meal can follow shortly thereafter. Colicky abdominal pain is a temporary discomfort and will disappear as soon as the patient returns to normal eating. Teach the patient to use throat lozenges or warm saline gargles to relieve soreness in the throat.

Before discharge, instruct the patient to notify the physician of any symptoms of abdominal pain, fever, nausea, or vomiting that are severe or prolonged.

⊙ **COMPLICATION ALERT** ⊙ Complications can appear within hours or even a day or two after the test. Because pancreatitis and bacterial infection in the biliary tract are the most common events, the nurse assesses for moderate to acute epigastric pain, nausea and vomiting, abdominal distension, fever, chills, and jaundice. Bleeding and perforation can also occur and the abdomen is assessed for ecchymosis (left flank and umbilical area), a distended, board-like abdomen, and melena. The patient may develop shock, dyspnea, and cardiac arrhythmia.

ENZYMES AND ISOENZYMES, CARDIAC • SERUM

NORMAL VALUES

CREATINE PHOSPHOKINASE (CPK) OR CREATINE KINASE (CK)
Adult male: 5–35 µg/ml
20–170 IU/L
<90 U/L
5–55 mU/ml
Adult female: 5–25 µg/ml
10–135 IU/L
<80 U/L
5–35 mU/ml
Male child: 0–70 IU/L
Female child: 0–50 IU/L
Newborn: 65–580 IU/L
10–200 U/L

NORMAL VALUES

CPK ISOENZYMES
CPK-MM (skeletal muscles): 90–97% of total CPK *or* SI 0.90–0.97 (fraction of total CPK)
CPK-MB (heart): 0–6% of total CPK *or* SI 0.00–0.06% (fraction of total CPK)
CPK-BB (brain): Trace or 0% of total CPK *or* SI trace or 0.00 (fraction of total CPK)

ASPARTATE AMINOTRANSFERASE (AST) OR SERUM GLUTAMIC OXALOACETIC TRANSAMINASE
Adult: 8–20 U/L
Older adult
Male: 11–26 U/L
Female: 10–20 U/L
Child (< 5 years): 19–28 U/L
Infant: 15–60 U/L
Newborn: 16–72 U/L

LACTIC ACID DEHYDROGENASE (LDH):
60–120 U/ml (Wacker scale)
150–450 U/ml (Wroblewski–La Due scale)

LDH ISOENZYMES:
70–200 IU/L
LDH_1:   Heart, red blood cells
14–26% *or* SI 0.14–0.26 (fraction of total LDH)
LDH_2:   Reticuloendothelial cells and kidney
29–39% *or* SI 0.29–0.39 (fraction of total LDH)
LDH_3:   Lungs, lymphatics, spleen, and others
20–26% *or* S1 0.20–0.26 (fraction of total LDH)
LDH_4:   Kidney, placenta, and liver
8–16% *or* S1 0.08–0.16 (fraction of total LDH)
LDH_5:   Kidney, liver, and skeletal muscle
6–16% *or* S1 0.06–0.16 (fraction of total LDH)

SERUM ALPHAHYDROXYBUTYRATE DEHYDROGENASE:
50–250 U/L

Purpose of the Test

Cardiac enzyme and isoenzyme studies are used with clinical evaluation and electrocardiographic studies to diagnose myocardial injury.

Enzymes are complex compounds found in all tissues that speed up the biochemical reactions of the body. Damage to body tissue causes release of enzymes from injured cells into the serum. Enzymes may be common to more than one type of tissue. Elevated serum levels of enzymes reflect tissue damage, but since the enzymes are not specific, patterns of enzyme elevations are used to determine myocardial tissue damage. Isoenzymes refer to the various forms of an enzyme, which differ chemically, physically, or immunologically, or a combination, but catalyze the same reaction.

Procedure

A venipuncture is necessary to obtain 5 to 10 ml of blood in a red-topped tube.

The cardiac enzyme protocol usually consists of CPK and its isoenzymes being collected three times, every 8 hours, after the onset of cardiac symptoms. CPK, CPK isoenzymes, LDH, LDH isoenzymes, and AST determinations are usually ordered at the onset of symptoms and thereafter every 24 hours three times.

✓ QUALITY CONTROL
Cardiac enzyme protocols require that isoenzymes be determined at certain frequencies and times. The nurse needs to coordinate the collection of the specimen to ensure accuracy of diagnosis and identification of possible extension of the infarction.

Findings

Multiple diagnoses cause changes in enzyme levels, as they are found in many body tissues. Because of this lack of specificity, enzymes alone do not establish diagnoses.

In diagnosing myocardial infarction, a pattern of enzyme changes *supports* the diagnosis. The first enzyme to rise is CPK. CPK levels begin to rise 6 hours after the infarction, peak in 18 hours, and return to normal in 2 to 3 days. CPK-MB levels rise within 3 to 6 hours after an infarction, peak in 12 to 24 hours, and return to normal in 12 to 48 hours. An increase in CPK-MB, expressed in a percentage of the total CPK, supports the diagnosis of myocardial damage. The percentage accepted as diagnostic of an infarction varies from laboratory to laboratory. If the CPK-MB level rises quickly and then drops quickly, myocardial contusion is suspected.

AST levels will begin to rise 6 to 10 hours after an infarction, peak in 24 to 48 hours, and return to normal after 4 to 6 days.

LDH elevations do not occur until 24 to 48 hours, peak in 3 to 4 days, and do not return to normal levels for 10 to 14 days after an infarction. LDH_2 levels are normally greater than LDH_1 levels. If LDH_1 levels become greater than those of LDH_2, it is called a "flipped" LDH and is indicative of a myocardial infarction. The flipped LDH is especially helpful if the person delayed seeking help when chest pain occurred.

Following a myocardial infarction, there is an elevation of the serum alpha-hydroxybutyrate level within 12 hours; it peaks in 48 to 72 hours and remains elevated for 1 to 3 weeks.

Because of their nonspecificity, other clinical problems may create changes in the enzyme levels. Common causes of these changes follow:

Increase in CPK

Amyotrophic lateral sclerosis
Biliary atresia
Burns
Cancers (some)
Cardiomyopathy
Central nervous system trauma, including cerebrovascular accident
Hypokalemia (severe)
Hypothermia
Hypothyroidism
Infarction (cerebral, bowel, myocardial)
Intramuscular injections
Muscular dystrophy
Myocarditis
Organ rejection
Pulmonary edema
Pulmonary embolism
Renal insufficiency or failure
Surgery

Decrease in CPK

Addison's disease
Anterior pituitary hyposecretion
Connective tissue disease
Alcoholic cirrhosis
Metastatic cancer
Steroid administration

Increase in AST

Cirrhosis
Congestive heart failure
Hepatitis
Myocardial infarction
Pericarditis
Pulmonary infarction
Reye's syndrome

Decrease in AST

Severe liver failure

Increase in LDH

Alcoholism
Anemia
Burns
Cancer

Decrease in LDH

Radiation therapy
Oxalates

Increase in LDH (cont.)

Cardiomyopathy
Cerebrovascular accident
Cirrhosis
Convulsions
Delirium tremens
Hepatitis
Hypothyroidism
Infectious mononucleosis
Codeine
Lithium carbonate
Meperidine
Morphine
Niacin
Pneumonia
Pulmonary infarction
Procainamide
Propranolol
Shock
Thyroid hormones
Ulcerative colitis

Increase in Serum Alpha-hydroxybutyrate Dehydrogenase

Anemia
Leukemia
Lymphoma
Malignant melanoma
Muscular dystrophy
Myocardial infarction
Nephrotic syndrome
Orthopedic hip surgery

Decrease in Serum Alpha-hydroxybutyrate Dehydrogenase

Clinically insignificant

Interfering Factors

CPK

Cardioversion
Drugs (alcohol, aspirin, halothane, lithium succinylcholine)
Muscle trauma
Recent vigorous exercise or massage
Surgery

AST

Drugs (acetaminophen, antituberculosis agents, aspirin, chlorpropamide, dicumarol, erythromycin, methyldopa, sulfonamides, vitamin A)

Muscle trauma

Not fasting

Strenuous fasting

LDH

Pregnancy

Prosthetic heart valves

Recent surgery

Nursing Implementation

• *Pretest*

Reassure the patient, who is usually frightened and having
chest pain, and may also be in denial.

Do *not* give intramuscular injections or perform repeated venipunctures, if possible, until all the initial enzyme studies are
completed.

Instruct the patient about the need to repeat blood sampling.

Determine if alcohol or drugs that affect results have been ingested.

• *During the Test*

If the tourniquet is in place too long, inaccurate results may
occur.

• *Posttest*

Nursing actions are similar to those for any venipuncture.

ERYTHROCYTE SEDIMENTATION RATE	• BLOOD

Synonyms: ESR, sed rate

N O R M A L   V A L U E S

ADULT <50 YEARS
Male: 0–15 mm/hour
Female: 0–20 mm/hour

ADULT >50 YEARS
Male: 0–20 mm/hour
Female: 0–30 mm/hour

CHILD:
0–10 mm/hour

Purpose of the Test

The erythrocyte sedimentation test is useful in identifying and monitoring disease activity in infectious, inflammatory, and neoplastic conditions. It is especially useful in rheumatic and collagen diseases.

Procedure

A purple- or blue-topped tube is used to collect 5 to 10 ml of venous blood.

✓ QUALITY CONTROL
Venipuncture technique must be smooth, with a blood flow that fills the vacuum tube readily. If the blood has excessive turbulence because of flawed technique, the hemolysis of erythrocytes will alter the test results.

Findings

Increase

Rheumatoid arthritis
Multiple myeloma
Rheumatic fever
Waldenström's macroglobulinemia
Inflammation
Anemia
Temporal arteritis
Pregnancy
Polymyalgia rheumatica

Decrease

Sickle cell anemia
Polycythemia
Spherocytosis
Hypofibrinogenemia

Interfering Factors

Anemia (ESR increases because there are fewer erythrocytes in the plasma)

Nursing Implementation

• *Pretest*

Since many medications, including salicylate, can alter laboratory values, list all medications taken by the patient on the requisition slip. In some cases, the medication may be withheld until after the test.

• *Posttest*

Ensure that the specimen is sent promptly to the laboratory. The specimen must be analyzed within 4 hours of collection.

ESOPHAGOGASTRODUODENOSCOPY (EGD)	• ENDOSCOPY

NORMAL VALUES

No abnormal structures or functions are observed in the esophagus, stomach, or duodenum.

Purpose of the Test

This diagnostic procedure is used to identify and biopsy tissue abnormality, determine the exact site and cause of upper gastrointestinal bleeding, evaluate the healing of gastric ulcers, evaluate the stomach and duodenum after gastric surgery, and to determine the cause of dysphagia, dyspepsia, gastric outlet obstruction, or epigastric pain.

Procedure

Once intravenous sedation is administered and the throat is anesthetized, the endoscope is used to visualize the inner surfaces of the esophagus, stomach, pylorus, and upper duodenum.

Tissue or cell samples are obtained for cytologic studies, as indicated.

Findings

Ulcers
Benign or malignant tumor
Diverticula
Esophageal stricture
Pyloric stenosis
Hiatal hernia inflammation
Mallory-Weiss tear
Varices

Interfering Factors

Failure to maintain a nothing-by-mouth status
Unstable or life-threatening cardiac or pulmonary condition
Known or suspected perforation of the stomach or intestine
Shock

Nursing Implementation

• *Pretest*

Schedule this test before or at least 2 days after an upper
   GI series so that the barium will not interfere with visualization.
Obtain a written consent.
Provide written posttest instructions now because temporary
   memory loss will occur after sedative administration.
When the procedure is to be performed in an ambulatory setting, someone must accompany the patient and provide
   transportation after discharge.
Instruct the patient to take nothing by mouth for 6 to 8 hours
   before the procedure.
Obtain the pretest coagulation profile, which includes prothrombin time, partial thromboplastin time, bleeding
   time, and platelet count. Place the results in the patient's
   chart.

On admission to the unit, obtain and record the vital signs.

Assist the patient with the removal and storage of eyeglasses, dentures, jewelry, hairpins, and clothing. A surgical gown is worn.

• During the Test

Position the patient on the examination table in the left lateral recumbent position. Apply the electronic monitoring devices for measurement of vital signs, ECG, and oxygen saturation.

Intravenous medication is given for relaxation and analgesia. Meperidine (Demerol) is often followed by diazepam (Valium) or midazolam (Versed). To prevent apnea, respiratory depression, or cardiac arrest, these medications are given slowly. Naloxone (Narcan) is kept on hand to reverse any respiratory depressive effect of meperidine, but it is ineffective against diazepam.

Oxygen delivered by nasal cannula will increase the patient's oxygen reserves and help prevent hypoxia.

Assist with the collection of specimens. Tissue samples are placed in a jar with preservative and labeled appropriately. The requisition slip includes the source of the tissue, the procedure, and the date.

✓ QUALITY CONTROL

On completion of the procedure, the laparoscope must be disassembled, thoroughly cleaned, and disinfected. Since the instrument is reused, these measures prevent transmission of infection.

• Posttest

Continue to assess the vital signs and level of consciousness until the patient is stable.

Review the posttest instructions, including the following: throat lozenges or saline gargle to relieve the discomfort in the throat, no driving for 12 hours, resumption of oral fluids and food after swallowing ability has returned.

⊘ **COMPLICATION ALERT** ⊘ If perforation or bleeding occurred during the procedure, the nurse must assess for hematemesis, melena, persistant pain (esophagus or epigastric area) and persistant dysphagia. Additionally, bacteremia and aspiration pneumonia may develop. The patient will develop chills, fever, malaise, a cough, or dyspnea.

ESTRADIOL (E₂) • SERUM

NORMAL VALUES

ADULT
Premenopausal female: 30–400 pg/ml *or* SI 110–1468 pmol/L
Postmenopausal female: 0–30 pg/ml *or* SI 0–110 pmol/L
Male: 10–50 pg/ml *or* SI 37–184 pmol/L

Purpose of the Test

The measurement of serum estradiol helps evaluate female infertility, menstrual irregularity, amenorrhea, or sexual precocity in the child. In the male, this test may be used to help evaluate a feminizing condition.

Procedure

A red-topped tube is used to collect 7 ml of venous blood.

Findings

Increase
Polycystic ovary
Adrenal tumor
Ovarian neoplasm or tumor
Gynecomastia
Hepatic cirrhosis
Hyperthyroidism

Decrease
Anorexia nervosa
Amenorrhea
Ovarian dysfunction
Ovarian hypofunction

Interfering Factors

Recent radioactive isotope scan

Nursing Implementation

- *Pretest*

Schedule this test before or at least 7 days after radioimmunoassay scan. The radioisotopes of the scan would interfere with the radioimmunoassay method of analysis.

- *Posttest*

To assist in the correct interpretation of the results, include the patient's age, phase of menstrual cycle, and the time that the test specimen was obtained.

Arrange for prompt transport of the blood to the laboratory.

> ✓ QUALITY CONTROL
> The serum must be extracted from the blood sample and frozen within 1 hour.

ESTRIOL, PREGNANCY (E₃) • SERUM, URINE

NORMAL VALUES

SERUM
(Teitz, 1995)
Weeks of gestation
28–30 weeks: 38–140 ng/ml *or* SI 132–486 nmol/L
32–34 weeks: 35–260 ng/ml *or* SI 121–902 nmol/L
36–38 weeks: 48–570 ng/ml *or* SI 167–1978 nmol/L
40 weeks: 95–460 ng/ml *or* SI 330–1596 nmol/L

URINE
(Teitz,1995)
First trimester: 0–800 μg/24 hours *or* SI 0–2776 nmol/24 hours
Second trimester: 800–12,000 μg/24 hours *or* SI 2776–41,640 nmol/24 hours
Third trimester: 5000–50,000 μg/24 hours *or* SI 17,350–173,500 nmol/24 hours

Purpose of the Test

In the later stages of pregnancy, the results of the serial estriol tests are used to evaluate fetal well-being and placental function, especially in the high-risk pregnancy.

Procedure

Serum

A red- or green-topped tube is used to obtain 5 to 7 ml of venous blood from the pregnant female.

Urine

A special laboratory container is used to collect a 24-hour specimen.

Findings

Decrease

Diabetes mellitus
Fetal growth retardation
Postmaturity
Fetal encephalopathy
Preeclampsia
Fetal adrenal aplasia
Erythroblastosis fetalis
Hemoglobinopathy
Intrauterine death

Interfering Factors

Recent radioisotope scan
Improper urine collection procedure
Failure to collect all urine in the test period
Failure to refrigerate the specimen
Improper labeling

Nursing Implementation

• *Pretest*

Urine

Provide both written and verbal instructions regarding the collection of the urine. These instructions must include the specific times for the collection period.

• *During the Test*

Urine

The first voided specimen of the morning is discarded and the urine collection period begins at 8 a.m.

The patient places all urine for 24 hours into the container. This includes the first voided specimen of the next morning.

Keep the specimen and container on ice or refrigerated during the collection period.

During the collection period, all urine is added to the container. If any urine spills or if a specimen is discarded accidentally, the test is invalidated. A new collection period is started on the following day.

- Posttest

Serum and Urine

Label the urine container (not the lid) with the patient's name and other appropriate identifying data. Include the time and date of the start and completion of the urine collection period.

Include the weeks of gestation on the requisition slip of each test.

Arrange for prompt delivery of the specimen to the laboratory.

✓ QUALITY CONTROL

For the serum specimen, the cells must be separated from the serum, and the serum is frozen immediately. The urine specimen must be refrigerated continuously until the urine is analyzed.

ESTROGEN-PROGESTERONE RECEPTOR ASSAY (ER-PgR)	• TISSUE BIOPSY

NORMAL VALUES

Negative: <3 fmol/mg cytosol protein *or* SI <3 nmol/kg cytosol protein
Borderline: 3–10 fmol/mg cytosol protein *or* SI 3–10 nmol/kg cytosol protein
Positive: >10 fmol/mg cytosol protein *or* SI >10 nmol/kg cytosol protein

Purpose of the Test

When breast tissue is malignant, the biopsy specimen is tested additionally to identify the presence of estrogen receptor sites and progesterone receptor sites. These two assays provide information regarding the potential effectiveness of hormonal therapy as a supplemental or palliative method of treatment of the malignancy. In each test, a value greater than 100 fmol/mg cytosol protein (SI >100 nmol/kg cytosol protein) is considered strongly positive and indicates the best potential for an effective treatment result.

Procedure

During a breast biopsy procedure, the tissue specimen is placed in a jar or waxed cardboard container. This jar or container is placed immediately in a larger container with ice.

Findings

Positive

Breast cancer that may respond to hormonal therapy

Interfering Factors

Use of a fixative on the tissue specimen
Delay in transport of the specimen
Inadequate tissue specimen

Nursing Implementation

- *Pretest*

On the requisition slip, identify the source and site of the tissue (left or right breast). See also the section on breast biopsy (pp. 44–46).

- *During the Test*

Ensure that the tissue is not fixed with a preservative. Place the container on ice.
Have the specimen sent immediately to the laboratory.

✓ QUALITY CONTROL
The specimen must be frozen within 15 to 30 minutes to prevent deterioration of the proteins at the receptor sites.

ESTROGEN, TOTAL   • URINE

NORMAL VALUES

Postmenopausal female: <20 µg/24 hours *or* SI 69 µmol/24 hours
Premenopausal female: 15–80 µg/24 hours *or* SI 52–277 µmol/24 hours
Male: 15–40 µg/24 hours *or* SI 52–139 µmol/24 hours
Child: <10 µg/24 hours *or* SI <35 µmol/24 hours

Purpose of the Test

The measurement of urinary estrogen is used to evaluate ovarian function, predict ovulation, determine the cause of amenorrhea, evaluate excess or decreased estrogen conditions, or help diagnose a testicular tumor.

Procedure

A special plastic collection bottle with a boric acid preservative is used to collect all urine for a 24-hour period.

Findings

Increase	*Decrease*
Male	Ovarian dysfunction
Testicular tumor	Pituitary gland hypofunction
Nonpregnant female	Ovarian insufficiency
Ovarian tumor	Adrenal gland hypofunction
Adrenocortical tumor	Menopause
Adrenocortical hyperplasia	Anorexia nervosa

Interfering Factors

Improper or incomplete collection of the urine.

Nursing Implementation

• *Pretest*

Provide both written and verbal instructions regarding the collection of urine.

• *During the Test*

The first voided specimen of the morning is discarded and the
    urine collection period begins at 8 a.m.
All urine for a 24-hour period is placed in the container. This
    includes the first voided specimen of the next morning.
Maintain the specimen and container on ice or refrigerated
    during the collection.

• *Posttest*

Label the urine container (not the lid) with the patient's
    name, the time and date of the start and completion of the
    urine collection period.
Write the patient's gender and age on the requisition slip. For
    the pregnant woman, also include the weeks of gestation.
Arrange for prompt delivery of the specimen to the laboratory.

✓ QUALITY CONTROL
The urine must be continuously refrigerated until it is analyzed.

F

FASTING BLOOD GLUCOSE	•	BLOOD, SERUM OR PLASMA

Synonyms: FBS, fasting blood sugar

N O R M A L   V A L U E S

Children (2 years–adult)
Whole blood: 60–110 mg/dl *or* SI 3.3–6.1 µmol/L
Plasma or serum: 70–120 mg/dl *or* SI 3.9–6.7 µmol/L
Elderly individuals: 80–150 mg/dl *or* SI 4.4–8.3 µmol/L
Children (<2 years): 60–100 mg/dl *or* SI 3.3–5.6 µmol/L
Infant: 40–90 mg/dl *or* SI 2.2–5.0 µmol/L
Neonate: 30–60 mg/dl *or* SI 1.7–3.3 µmol/L
With age, the norms for blood and plasma glucose levels are adjusted by 1 mg/dl per year after age 60.

Purpose of the Test

Fasting blood glucose is evaluated to diagnose and manage patients with diabetes mellitus. The fasting blood glucose level is also obtained as supportive data in many diagnoses, as metabolic factors will influence glucose use and storage. Certain therapies may be evaluated by checking the fasting blood glucose level, for example, hyperalimentation and exogenous glucocorticoid therapy.

One elevated fasting blood glucose level is not considered diagnostic but should be repeated. If a repeated fasting blood glucose level is elevated (>140 mg/dl), it supports the diagnosis of diabetes mellitus.

Procedure

After a 12-hour fast, venipuncture is performed to obtain 1 ml of blood in a red-topped tube for a plasma or serum sample or in a green-topped tube for a whole blood sample. Usually serum or plasma sampling is performed because these tests reflect glucose levels in interstitial tissue and are not affected by the hematocrit.

Findings

Increase	*Decrease*
Acromegaly	Addison's disease
Chronic pancreatitis	Advanced liver disease
Cushing's syndrome	Alcohol when fasting
Diabetes mellitus	Excessive exogenous insulin
Hyperthyroidism	Islet cell adenoma
Hyperosmolar coma	Leucine sensitivity
Pheochromocytoma	Malnutrition
Stress	

Interfering Factors

Noncompliance with fasting
Vigorous exercise
Stress
Medications (acetaminophen, arginine, benzodiazepines, beta-blockers, epinephrine, ethacrynic acid, furosemide, glucocorticoids, glucose intake, hypoglycemic agents, insulin, lithium, MAO inhibitors, oral contraceptives, phenothiazines, phenytoin, thiazide diuretics)

Nursing Implementation

The nurse's actions are similar to those in other venipuncture procedures.

• *Pretest*

Instruct the patient to fast for 12 hours before the blood is drawn.
Explain to the patient who is taking insulin or hypoglycemic agents to withhold the medication until after the blood is drawn.

✪ **COMPLICATION ALERT** ✪ Because a fasting blood glucose determination requires that the patient maintain a nothing-by-mouth status, hypoglycemia may occur. The nurse needs to assess for pallor, diaphoresis, tachycardia, palpitations, hunger, paresthesia, confusion, slurred speech, somnolence, convulsions, and coma.

- *Posttest*

Ensure that the patient receives food and medications that were withheld.

Send blood to the laboratory, as it needs to be centrifuged within 30 minutes for serum and plasma levels.

FAT, FECAL (STOOL FAT, QUANTITATIVE)	• FECES

NORMAL VALUES

Adult: 2–7 g/24 hours *or* SI 2–7 g/24 hours
Fat-free diet: < 4 g/24 hours
Child
0–6 years: <2 g/24 hours
Breast fed: <1 g/24 hours

Purpose of the Test

Fecal fat is used to identify steatorrhea and evaluate the ability to digest fat from dietary intake. Abnormal results support evidence of hepatobiliary, or pancreatic or small intestinal disease.

Procedure

For the 6 days of the test, the patient eats a standard, high-fat diet (100 g of fat per day). The collection of feces is done on days 4, 5, and 6 of the diet. All fecal matter in the 72-hour period is collected in a clean, heavy plastic, screw-capped container and kept refrigerated.

Findings

Increase

Pancreatic insufficiency
Obstruction or resection
Cystic fibrosis
Chronic pancreatitis
Regional enteritis
Celiac disease

Increase (cont.)

Tropical sprue
Radiation enteritis
Gastroduodenal fistula
Extensive small bowel resection
Dumping syndrome
Biliary tract obstruction
Scleroderma
Liver cirrhosis
Impaired hepatic function

Interfering Factors

Use of improper collecting container
Contamination of the sample
Failure to follow the dietary prescription
Omission of any specimen
Ingestion of alcohol or use of mineral oil during the test

Nursing Implementation

• *Pretest*

Instruct the patient to follow the prescribed diet for 3 days before and 3 days during the test. Ingestion of alcohol is omitted for 24 hours before collection and during the 3 days of
collection.
No use of laxatives or cathartics is permitted.
Instruct the patient as to proper collection procedure, including the correct type of container.

> ✓ QUALITY CONTROL
> Improper containers include coffee cans, paper cartons, waxed
> containers, or plastic bags. The specimen must be free of urine,
> toilet paper, tongue depressors, and plastic spoons.

• *During the Test*

Ensure that the specimen is refrigerated for the entire collection
period and until it is transported to the laboratory.

• *Posttest*

Write the time and date for the start and finish of the collection
period on the container label and requisition slip.

FIBRINOGEN (FACTOR I)   •   PLASMA

N O R M A L   V A L U E S

Adult: 200–400 mg/dl or SI 2–4 g/L

Purpose of the Test

Fibrinogen, a coagulation protein, is a vital component of clot formation. When fibrinogen is excessive, the patient may form a thrombus or embolus. With a severely reduced level, the patient is prone to hemorrhage. The fibrinogen test is used to help diagnose bleeding disorders, including afibrinogenemia, DIC, and fibrinolysis.

Procedure

A blue-topped tube with sodium citrate is used to obtain 4.5 ml of venous blood. As an alternative, a heelstick, earlobe, or finger puncture may be used to collect capillary blood in siliconized sodium citrate micropipettes.

✓ QUALITY CONTROL
The tube must be filled with blood. If filling is incomplete, the increased proportion of sodium citrate will cause a false elevation of the test result. To mix the sodium citrate with the blood, the specimen tube is tilted gently from side to side, 5 to 10 times. When multiple specimens are drawn, the fibrinogen test specimen is obtained last, using double-tube technique. A 1- to 2-ml blood sample is obtained and discarded; the blue-topped tube is then used to collect the test sample. To prevent hemolysis and a false decrease in the test result, venipuncture technique must be smooth, with a blood flow that fills the vacuum tube readily.

Findings

Increase	*Decrease*
Sepsis-infection	Hereditary afibrinogenemia
Malignancy	Hypofibrinogenemia
Inflammation	Severe liver disease
Traumatic injury	DIC

Interfering Factors

Heparinization
Pregnancy (third trimester)
Recent surgery
Inadequate amount of specimen
Hemolysis
Coagulation of the specimen

Nursing Implementation

- *Pretest*

For the patient who receives intermittent doses of heparin, schedule the test at least 1 hour after heparin dose is administered.

- *Posttest*

Arrange for prompt transport of the specimen to the laboratory.

> ✓ QUALITY CONTROL
> The results are invalid with a clotted specimen or a time delay of greater than 1 hour before the cells are separated from the plasma.

FIBRIN SPLIT PRODUCTS (FSP, FDP, FBP)   • PLASMA

N O R M A L   V A L U E S

<10 µg/ml *or* SI <10 mg/L

Purpose of the Test

In the normal process of fibrinolysis or the dissolving of a clot, the end product is called fibrin split product, fibrin degradation product, or fibrin breakdown product. When clotting and breakdown is excessive, the serum level rises. The possible panic level of greater than 40 µg/ml indicates that DIC is the probable cause.

This test is used to help diagnose DIC and to monitor fibrinolytic therapy. It may be used in the study of disorders that produce clot formation and lysis of the clot.

Procedure

A special tube for fibrin split products is used to collect 2 ml of venous blood. The tube, obtained from the coagulation laboratory, contains thrombin and an antifibrinolytic agent.

✓ QUALITY CONTROL
Once the blood is drawn, the tube is tilted from side to side
5 to 10 times to mix the blood with the clotting agents. The
blood will coagulate.

Findings

Increase

DIC
Primary or secondary fibrinolysis
Myocardial infarction
Pulmonary embolus
Malignancy
Liver disease
Infection or inflammation

Interfering Factors

Improper collection or storage procedure

Nursing Implementation

- *Posttest*

Arrange for prompt transport of the specimen to the laboratory.

✓ QUALITY CONTROL
For analysis, the blood must clot in the tube for 30 minutes; the
sample is then centrifuged to separate the cells from the serum.

FOLLICLE STIMULATING HORMONE (FSH)	• SERUM, URINE

N O R M A L   V A L U E S

SERUM
Adult male: 1–7 mU/ml *or* SI: 1–7 U/L
Adult female
Follicular and luteal phases: 1–9 mU/ml *or* SI 1–9 U/L
Midcycle peak: 6–26 mU/ml *or* SI 6–26 U/L
Postmenopausal phase: 30–118 mU/ml *or* SI 30–118 U/L
Child 6 months–10 years: <1–3 mU/ml *or* SI <1–3 U/L

URINE
Adult male: 4–18 U/24 hours *or* SI 4–18 U/24 hours
Adult female
Follicular phase: 3–12 U/24 hours *or* SI 3–12 U/24 hours
Midcycle peak: 8–60 U/24 hours *or* SI 8–60 U/24 hours
Child 1–8 years
Male: 0.5–4.5 U/24 hours *or* SI 0.5–4.5 U/24 hours
Female: 0.5–4 U/24 hours *or* SI 0.5–4 U/24 hours

Purpose of the Test

The measurement of FSH is used to help diagnose gonadal dysfunction or failure, including delayed sexual maturation, menstrual disturbance, or amenorrhea. It is also used to evaluate infertility in the female and testicular dysfunction in the male.

The urinary test is used for children with precocious puberty and to identify the time of ovulation when in vitro fertilization is planned.

Procedure

Serum

A red- or green-topped tube is used to collect 5 to 7 ml of venous blood.

> ✓ QUALITY CONTROL
> Venipuncture technique must be smooth, with a blood flow that fills the vacuum tube readily. If the blood has excessive turbulence because of flawed venipuncture technique, the hemolysis of the erythrocytes will alter the test results.

Urine

A large plastic urine container is used to collect all urine for 24 hours.

Findings

Increase	*Decrease*
Primary testicular failure	Polycystic disease of the ovary
Orchitis	Hypofunction of anterior pituitary or hypothalamus
Castration	

Idiopathic precocious puberty
Ovarian agenesis
Menopause
Central nervous system lesion

Anorexia nervosa
Adrenal tumor
Congenital adrenal hypo-
    plasia
Sickle cell disease

Interfering Factors

Recent radioactive isotope scan
Hemolysis
Incomplete collection of urine

Nursing Implementation

• *Pretest*

Schedule this test before or 1 to 7 days after a nuclear scan examination.

Urine

Provide both written and verbal instructions regarding the collection procedure.

• *During the Test*

The first voided specimen of the morning is discarded, and
    the urine collection period begins at 8 a.m.
All urine is collected for 24 hours and placed in the container.
    This includes the first voided specimen of the next morn-
    ing.
Maintain the specimen and container on ice or refrigerate dur-
    ing the collection period.

• *Posttest*

Urine

On the requisition slip, write the time and date of the start and
completion of the test.

Serum and Urine

For the female, include the date of the last menstrual period
    on the requisition slip.

Because of refrigeration needs, deliver the specimen to the laboratory, without delay.

FREE THYROXINE • SERUM

Synonym: FT$_4$

NORMAL VALUES

0.9–1.7 mg/dl *or* SI 11.5–21.8 nmol/L

Purpose of the Test

The majority of thyroxine is carried by thyroid-binding globulin, albumin, and prealbumin. It is free and unbound thyroxine, which is biologically active and converts to triiodothyronine (T$_3$) in the peripheral circulation. The ability to measure free thyroxine has replaced a classic test called protein-bound iodine.

Free thyroxine is used to diagnose hyper- and hypothyroidism. It is especially helpful when there is abnormal thyroxine-binding globulin levels.

Procedure

Venipuncture is performed to collect 1 ml of blood in a red-topped tube. Laboratory procedures vary in assessing free thyroxine. If RIA is performed, albumin levels and a radionuclide scan within 7 days will affect the results.

Findings

Increase

Acute psychiatric disorder
Hyperthyroidism

Decrease

Anorexia nervosa
Hypothyroidism

Interfering Factors

Medications

Carbamazepine
Exogenous thyroid therapy
Heparin
Phenytoin
Salicylates

Nursing Implementation

The nurse takes actions similar to those taken in other venipuncture procedures.

FREE TRIIODOTHYRONINE • SERUM

Synonym: FT$_3$

NORMAL VALUES

0.2–0.52 mg/dl *or* SI 3–8 nmol/L

Purpose of the Test

Triiodothyronine is a hormone secreted by the thyroid gland. Most of the hormone is bound to thyroid-binding globulin. Some triiodothyronine is in the free state, that is, unbound. The unbound or free triiodothyronine is the biologically active form of the hormone.

Free triiodothyronine is used to diagnose hyper- and hypothyroidism.

Procedure

Venipuncture is performed to collect a 1-ml specimen in a red-topped tube. Laboratory methods to assess free triiodothyronine vary. If RIA is used, albumin levels and a radionuclide scan within 7 days will affect results.

Findings

Increase	*Decrease*
Hyperthyroidism	Hypothyroidism

Interfering Factors

Exogenous thyroid therapy

Nursing Implementation

Nursing actions resemble those of other venipuncture procedures.

G

• RADIOGRAPHY

NORMAL VALUES

The gallbladder and biliary ductal system is patent, with no evidence of stones, obstruction, or other abnormality.

Purpose of the Test

Gallbladder radiography is used to visualize the storage and excretion functions of the gallbladder and biliary ductal system. The x-rays provide visualization of stones and other causes of obstruction.

Procedure

Iodine-based, radiopaque contrast material is given orally or intravenously. Initial x-rays are taken of the biliary structures and the storage ability of the gallbladder. After a fatty substance is given orally or intravenously, additional x-rays are taken at intervals to visualize the emptying of the gallbladder and biliary ducts.

Findings

Stone(s) in the gallbladder
Cystic duct or common duct
Inflammatory disease of the gallbladder
Nonfunctional gallbladder
Polyps or benign tumors of the biliary ducts

Interfering Factors

Retained barium in the intestine
Failure to maintain a fat-free diet and nothing-by-mouth status
  before the test

Impaired hepatic function
Biliary obstruction and jaundice
Pregnancy (first trimester)

Nursing Implementation

• *Pretest*

Schedule this test before any required barium tests.

> ✓ QUALITY CONTROL
> Retained barium in the intestinal tract will obscure the view of the gallbladder and biliary tree.

Question the patient for any history of allergy to iodine, seafood, or previous allergic reaction during a diagnostic test that used an iodine-based dye.

Obtain a written consent.

Instruct the patient regarding pretest procedure.

Cholecystography, Oral

1. To cleanse the bowel of fecal matter and gas, the patient takes two bisacodyl (Ducolax) tablets on the morning of the day before the test.
2. The patient must eat a fat-free meal the night before the test, with no further intake of food or beverages, except water.
3. Two or three hours after dinner, the patient begins to take the 6 tablets of ionopaque acid (Telepaque), with 8 oz of water. One tablet is taken every 5 minutes until all 6 are ingested. After taking the contrast, any diarrhea or vomiting is reported to the physician.

> ✓ QUALITY CONTROL
> If the patient has less than the required dose of contrast medium there will be inadequate visualization of gallbladder and ducts.

4. The patient may continue to drink water, as desired until midnight and is completely nothing-by-mouth thereafter.
5. In the early morning, a saline enema may be required.

Cholangiography, Intravenous

1. Instruct the patient about pretest preparation, including the above method of bowel cleansing and the discontinuation of all food and fluid after midnight on the night before the test.

2. Advise the patient that a sensation of warmth and flushing of the skin may be felt at the time of the injection of the contrast medium. Reassure the patient that this is a common sensation and will only last for a short while.

✪ **COMPLICATION ALERT** ✪ Mild to severe allergic reaction to iodine may occur. The nurse should assess for hives, swelling, apprehension, and respiratory difficulty as early signs of a problem. A more severe response includes acute respiratory distress and shock.

GAMMA GLUTAMYL TRANSFERASE (GGT) • SERUM

NORMAL VALUES

Male (16–60 years): 7–47 IU/L or SI 0.12–0.80 µKat/L
Female (16–60 years): 4–25 U/L or SI 0.07–0.43 µKat/L

Purpose of the Test

The gamma glutamyl transferase test is used to detect hepatobiliary disease with intrahepatic or posthepatic biliary obstruction. It is also used to diagnose and evaluate chronic alcoholic liver disease.

Procedure

A red- or green-topped sterile tube is used to collect 5 to 10 ml of venous blood.

Findings

Increase	*Decrease*
Obstructive biliary or liver disease	Hypothyroidism
Cancer of the pancreas or liver	
Hepatitis	
Cirrhosis	
Systemic lupus erythematosus	

Infectious mononucleosis
Acute pancreatitis
Hyperthyroidism

Interfering Factors

Intake of alcohol within 60 hours before the test
Use of barbiturates
Phenytoin or oral contraceptives
Failure to maintain nothing-by-mouth status

Nursing Implementation

- *Pretest*

Instruct the patient to abstain from alcohol for 72 hours prior
to the test.

Inform the patient to fast from food and fluids for 12 hours
before the test.

Inform the physician or laboratory of the use of those medications that would interfere with the results. Patients who must
maintain their medication schedule should not eliminate
the pills in the pretest period.

GASTRIN • SERUM

NORMAL VALUES

Adult (16–60 years): 25–90 pg/ml *or* SI 25–90 ng/ml
Child: <10–125 pg/ml *or* SI <10–125 ng/L

Purpose of the Test

The two gastrins are peptides that stimulate the production of
gastric acid and the secretion of pepsin and intrinsic factor. Serum gastrin is helpful in the diagnosis of Zollinger-Ellison syndrome and pernicious anemia.

Procedure

A red-topped tube without anticoagulant is used to collect 5 to 10 ml of venous blood.

Findings

Increase	*Decrease*
Zollinger-Ellison syndrome	Antrectomy with vagotomy surgery
Pernicious anemia	Hypothyroidism
Chronic atrophic gastritis	
Gastric ulcer	
Pyloric obstruction	
Chronic renal failure	
Gastric cancer	

Interfering Factors

Failure to fast from food
Recent radioisotope administration
Gastroscopy

Nursing Implementation

- *Pretest*

Schedule this test before gastroscopy and any radioisotope procedures.

Instruct the patient to discontinue all food intake for at least 12 hours before the test.

✓ QUALITY CONTROL
Recent ingestion of protein would cause an elevation of the serum gastrin level.

- *Posttest*

Ensure that the specimen is sent to the laboratory without delay.

✓ QUALITY CONTROL
Gastrin is unstable at room temperature. Delay will invalidate the results. In the laboratory, the serum is separated out by refrigerated centrifuge and the specimen is frozen immediately.

GATED BLOOD POOL STUDIES	•	RADIONUCLIDE IMAGING

Synonyms: Technetium-99 ventriculography, MUGA, multiple gated acquisition angiography

N O R M A L   V A L U E S

Normal wall motion
Ejection fraction = 55–75%
Response to exercise—increase in ejection fraction >5%

Purpose of the Test

A gated blood pool scan is a noninvasive method of assessing myocardial function, particularly wall motion of the left ventricle. It also permits evaluation of left ventricular ejection without invasive catheterization.

Procedure

The procedure for the gated pool study is similar to that for myocardial imaging. The red blood cells are tagged with technetium-99m pyrophosphate, a gamma-emitting radionuclide. Since the bound technetium cannot diffuse through cell membranes, it remains in the blood. Its emissions are more concentrated in body cavities with large blood volumes, including the heart chambers.

During the procedure, the patient is monitored with a cardiac monitor, and the ECG is synchronized with the imaging equipment. Multiple images can be obtained. Results usually report the "first pass," which analyzes the radiotracing during the initial flow through the heart. In addition, a "gated" analysis is performed, which reports cardiac chamber responses of 200 to 300 cardiac cycles. Since left ventricular size can be measured at the end of diastole and systole, the ventricular ejection fraction can be measured. After a gated analysis, the patient may or may not be reassessed with exercise stress testing.

Findings

Hypokinesis: slightly diminished wall motion
Akinesis: absence of wall motion
Dyskinesia: paradoxical wall motion or bulging
Decreased ejection fraction

Nursing Implementation

See section on nuclear imaging and stress testing (pp. 233–235).

GENITAL CULTURE • SECRETIONS

NORMAL VALUES

Negative; normal flora present

Purpose of the Test

The genital culture is used to identify the pathogenic organism that causes abnormal discharge and inflammation of the vagina or male urethra.

Procedure

Female. With the assistance of a speculum, a sterile swab or wire loop is inserted into the cervical canal to obtain secretions or endocervical cell scrapings.

Male. A sterile cotton swab is used to collect secretions from the penile discharge. The physician may insert a wire loop into the urethra to obtain cell scrapings.

Chancroid. The base of the genital ulcer is irrigated with saline. The fluid is aspirated with a sterile pipette or a moist, sterile cotton swab.

Herpes simplex. A sterile cotton swab is used to remove epithelial cells from the base of fresh lesions. Fluid from vesicles may also be obtained by aspiration with a sterile pipette.

For any of these procedures, a sterile culture tube is used to receive cell scrapings or fluid aspirate.

Findings

Positive

Gonorrhea (*Neisseria gonorrhoeae*)
Nonspecific vaginitis (*Candida albicans, Gardnerella vaginalis*)
Genital herpes (herpes simplex virus)
Trichomoniasis (*Trichomonas vaginalis*)
Toxic shock syndrome (*Staphylococcus aureus*)

Chlamydia (*Chlamydia trachomatis*)
Chancroid (*Haemophilus ducreyi*)
Giardiasis (*Giardia lamblia*)
Genital warts (human papillomavirus)

Interfering Factors

Recent urination
Recent douching
Improper collection technique
Contamination of the specimen
Antibiotic administration

Nursing Implementation

• *Pretest*

Instruct the patient as follows.
   Male: Do not urinate within 1 hour of the test.
   Female: Do not douche for 24 hours before the test.
Inquire about any current use of antibiotics. The culture
   should be performed before any antibiotic therapy is
   started.

• *During the Test*

Place the male in the supine position. The female is placed in
   the lithotomy position.
Provide emotional support to the patient during the collection
   of the specimen. For the female, the procedure may produce mild apprehension or discomfort. The male may experience nausea, sweating, fainting, or weakness as the wire
   loop or swab is inserted into the urethra.
Place the specimen into the culture tube.

• *Posttest*

The requisition slip should identify the source of the specimen, the patient's name and age, the clinical diagnosis, the
   time and date of the specimen collection, and any current
   antibiotic therapy.
Arrange for transport of the specimen to the laboratory within
   2 hours. It must not be refrigerated.
Instruct the patient to abstain from sexual contact until the results are known and the infection is treated and cured.

When the culture is positive for a sexually transmitted disease, instruct the patient to inform all sexual partners of the test results. Sexual contacts are advised to undergo testing. Gonorrhea is reported to the state health department.

With gonorrheal infection, instruct the patient to have the culture repeated 1 week after the completion of antibiotic therapy.

GLUCAGON • PLASMA

N O R M A L   V A L U E S

50–100 pg/ml *or* SI 25 ng/L

Purpose of the Test

Glucagon is produced and secreted by the A cells of the islets of Langerhans of the pancreas. Glucagon stimulates the breakdown of stored glycogen and maintains gluconeogenesis. Glucagon is secreted in response to hypoglycemia, helping to meet glucose needs of tissues between intakes of food.

Glucagon levels are assessed in suspected pancreatic tumors, chronic pancreatitis, and familial hyperglucagonemia.

Procedure

Venipuncture is performed to obtain 7 ml of blood in a lavender-topped tube with EDTA. The specimen is placed on ice and sent to the laboratory immediately to be centrifuged.

Findings

Increase	*Decrease*
Acute pancreatitis	Chronic pancreatitis
Diabetic ketoacidosis	High fatty acid levels
Glucagonoma	Hyperglycemia
Hypoglycemia	Insulinoma
Parasympathetic stimulation	
Pheochromocytoma	
Renal failure	
Stress	
Sympathetic stimulation	

Interfering Factors

Stress
Prolonged fasting
Radioactive scan within 2 days
Medications (catecholamines, insulin, glucocorticoids)

Nursing Implementation

The nurse takes actions similar to those used in other venipuncture procedures.

• *Pretest*

Instruct the patient to fast for 10 to 12 hours before blood is drawn.

Explain to the patient the need to rest for 30 minutes before the test.

Take a medication history and determine if any interfering drugs should be withheld.

Schedule any radioactive scans after the glucagon determination is obtained.

Place specimen on ice and send to laboratory immediately. (Not all laboratories require the specimen to be placed on ice.)

• *Posttest*

The patient can resume a normal diet and medication regimen.

GLUCOSE, CAPILLARY • WHOLE BLOOD

Synonyms: Self-blood glucose monitoring (SBGM), bedside glucose monitoring (BGM)

NORMAL VALUES

60–110 mg/dl *or* SI 3.3–6.1 µmol/L

Purpose of the Test

Capillary glucose monitoring is carried out to assess and manage patients with diabetes mellitus. It may be used in hospitals to monitor other hyperglycemic patients, such as those patients on hyperalimentation or high-dose glucocorticoid therapy. Capillary glucose evaluation is *not* used to diagnose diabetes mellitus, but it may indicate a need to perform a glucose tolerance test.

For insulin-dependent (IDDM) and noninsulin dependent (NIDDM) diabetics, regular capillary glucose testing will produce greater control with more effective long-term treatment. Capillary glucose testing can help the diabetic maintain control during periods of stress; for example, during illness, pregnancy, and surgery. Usually, the patient with IDDM will monitor the capillary glucose level before each meal and at bedtime. The patient with noninsulin dependent diabetes (NIDDM) usually monitors the capillary glucose twice a day—before breakfast and 2 hours after dinner. NIDDM patients can check their glucose level 2 hours after they eat to see how specific foods affect it and modify their intake by an objective measurement.

Procedure

With a lancet, a fingerstick is carried out, and a drop of blood is dropped onto a reagent strip. The intensity of the color change is proportional to the amount of glucose in the blood. The darker the color, the higher the glucose concentration. The color change is assessed visually by comparing it to a color chart or by the blood glucose meter. The meter may read the strip by the process of refractance photometry or by electrochemical technology. Either method will provide a digital read-out of the glucose level.

Nursing Implementation

Nurses need to teach their patients how to monitor capillary glucose, including how to use and care for the glucose meter and reagent strips and how to check the reliability of the meter. This information needs to be reinforced periodically.

There are many different glucose meters on the market. It is *essential* to follow the manufacturers' guidelines for their use. In addition, there are a number of lancing devices available.

• *Pretest*

✓ QUALITY CONTROL
Glucose meters should be checked daily in hospitals and once a week or when opening a new vial of strips at home with quality control solution containing a known amount of dissolved glucose in water. The meter should also be tested if the meter is dropped or the meter reading does not correlate with clinical assessments.

✓ QUALITY CONTROL
When a fasting blood glucose determination is obtained, a capillary glucose level can also be obtained and the two measures compared. A variance of less than 15% is acceptable.

If the battery in the meter has worn out, recalibrate the meter with the plastic calibration strip provided in the reagent vial according to the manufacturer's guidelines.

Check the code number on the glucose meter and on the reagent strip to ensure that they are the same. Check the expiration date on the reagent strip container and discard outdated strips.

Wear gloves for this procedure, as blood contact is possible.

• *During the Test*

Instruct the patient to wash their hands in warm water and soap. The warm water will help dilate the vessels.

Hospital protocol may require the patient's finger to be wiped with an alcohol swab (this is usually not done in the home). If alcohol is used, it must be allowed to dry out or it will affect the results and increase the painfulness of the procedure.

Have the reagent strip on hand, and puncture the skin. The puncture site should be on the side of the fingertip. The middle of the fingertip is more sensitive to pain, and the side has more capillaries. Instruct the patient to rotate sites.

Milk the fingertip toward the puncture site until a large drop of blood forms.

Let the drop of blood fall on the reagent strip so that the entire pad at the tip is covered with blood. Do not smear the blood or try to add another drop.

Time when to wipe the strip and when to insert the strip into the meter, if required according to the manufacturer's guidelines. Timing is essential for accurate measurement.

Some manufacturers require a cotton ball be used to wipe the reagent strip.

Insert the strip into the meter. Read and document the results.

Instruct the patient on how to dispose of the lancet in a heavy plastic container; for example, an empty detergent bottle.

• *Posttest*

Administer insulin as ordered.

Instruct the patient to keep an accurate record of the glucose
  level and insulin replacement. This record should be
  brought to the physician, diabetic nurse specialist, or clinic
  on the next visit.

GLUCOSE TOLERANCE TEST • PLASMA

Synonyms: GTT, OGTT, IVGTT

NORMAL VALUES

Baseline FBS: 70–105 mg/dl *or* SI 3.9–5.8 µmol/L
30-minute BS: 110–170 mg/dl *or* SI 6.1–9.4 µmol/L
60-minute BS: 120–170 mg/dl *or* SI 6.7–9.4 µmol/L
90-minute BS: 100–140 mg/dl *or* SI 5.6–7.8 µmol/L
120-minute BS: 70–120 mg/dl *or* SI 3.9–6.7 µmol/L

Purpose of the Test

Fasting blood glucose levels are usually, if repeated, adequate to
diagnose diabetes mellitus if the plasma glucose level is more
than 140 mg/dl. However, if the fasting blood glucose level is
between 120 and 140 mg/dl and additional clinical indications
make diabetes mellitus likely, an *oral glucose tolerance test* (OGTT)
may be performed.

The *intravenous glucose tolerance test* (IVGTT) is similar to the
OGTT. It is usually ordered when the patient has a problem with
gastrointestinal absorption. It is not preferable to the OGTT because it bypasses normal glucose absorption and, therefore, normal changes in gastrointestinal hormones. Patient preparation
for the IVGGT is the same as that for the OGTT, except that the
glucose load (0.5 gm/kg of ideal body weight) is given intravenously over 2 to 3 minutes. The fasting blood glucose levels after
the IVGTT are similar to those after an OGTT, except that the 30-
minute ingestion fasting blood glucose level tends to be higher.

Procedure

After the ingestion of a glucose load, venous blood samplings for
plasma glucose are obtained at the time of ingestion and then
at 30, 60, 90, and 120 minutes after the glucose load is given.

Findings

The OGTT confirms the diagnosis of diabetes mellitus if the 2-hour blood glucose level is greater than 200 mg/dl and at least one other blood glucose determination is greater than 200 mg/dl. Blood glucose levels between the diagnostic criteria and normal values are called "impaired glucose tolerance."

Interfering Factors

Noncompliance with dietary and fasting requirements
Alcohol ingestion
Being bedridden
Cushing's syndrome or Cushing's disease
Infection
Malabsorption syndrome
Malnutrition
Pregnancy
Severe stress
Medications (amphetamines, arginine, beta-adrenergic blockers, diuretics, epinephrine, glucocorticoids, glucose administered intravenously, insulin, lithium, oral contraceptives, oral hypoglycemic agents, phenothiazines, phenytoin, salicylates)

Nursing Implementation for OGTT

• *Pretest*

Instruct the patient to take in at least 150 to 250 g of carbohydrates per day for 3 days before the test to optimize insulin secretion.

Instruct the patient not to drink or eat for 8 hours before the test begins. The patient is also instructed to avoid stimulants and not to smoke or perform any unusual activity for 8 hours before the test.

Take a medication history to determine if any interfering drugs are being taken. Check with the prescriber to determine if medications should be withheld. Oral hypoglycemic agents are withheld for 2 weeks before an OGTT is performed.

Question the patient regarding any recent acute illnesses. The OGTT should be delayed for at least 2 weeks after an acute illness.

- *During the Test*

A fasting blood glucose determination is performed (usually in the early morning between 7 and 9 a.m.).

Within 5 minutes of obtaining the baseline fasting blood glucose level, the patient drinks 75 g of glucose in 300 ml of water. Children are given 1.5 g of glucose per kilogram of ideal body weight. The glucose solution should be ingested within 5 minutes.

Venipunctures are performed to obtain blood glucose readings at 30, 60, 90, and 120 minutes after the glucose solution is ingested. If a hypoglycemic reaction is suspected, a 3-hour blood specimen is obtained.

Observe the patient for a hyper- or hypoglycemic reaction.

The patient may drink water during the collection period.

- *Posttest*

The patient resumes taking medications that were withheld.
A normal diet and activity level are resumed.

GLUCOSE, URINARY • URINE

Synonyms: None

N O R M A L   V A L U E S
No glucose present

Purpose of the Test

When capillary glucose monitoring is not possible, urinary glucose is measured to determine insulin and dietary requirements of patients with diabetes mellitus.

Procedure

Two methods are commonly used to check for urinary glucose: copper reduction tests (Clinitest tablets) or the dipstick method. The latter is more frequently used at home.

Findings

Glucosuria may be due to diabetes mellitus, chronic renal failure, Cushing's syndrome, thyroid disorders, Fanconi's syndrome, hyperalimentation, or pregnancy.

Interfering Factors

Failure to use fresh urine

Urine heavily contaminated with bacteria

Clinitest tablet or dipstick was exposed to air, light, heat, or moisture

Medications (partial listing: acetylsalicylic acid, chloral hydrate, glucocorticoids, isoniazid, levodopa, lithium, methyldopa, penicillin G, probenecid, salicylates, streptomycin, tetramycin, thiazide diuretics)

Nursing Implementation

Since this test is used for self-monitoring, patient education is an essential part of the nursing role.

- *Pretest*

Instruct the patient on the double-void technique.

Explain to the patient the need to collect the specimen in a clean container.

With the Clinitest tablets, heat is created by the chemical action. Warn the patient not to hold the test tube in the hand after dropping the tablet into it.

- *During the Test*

With the Clinitest Tablet

Add to a clean, dry test tube five drops of urine and ten drops of water and then drop a Clinitest tablet into the test tube.

Compare the color change of the urine with the color chart that comes with the tablets.

Record results.

With Dipstick Method (Clinistix, Diastix, Tes-Tape)

The dipstick is dipped in urine. The waiting time is indicated by the manufacturer.

Compare color change with chart provided.

Record results.

- *Posttest*

Clean equipment with soap and water, and rinse thoroughly.

Store tablets and dipstick in dry, cool place in their original containers.

Document results on flow sheet.
Adjust insulin dosage as ordered based on the results.

GLYCOSYLATED HEMOGLOBIN ASSAY • BLOOD

Synonyms: Glycohemoglobin, GHB, hemoglobin A_1

N O R M A L   V A L U E S

GLYCOSYLATED HEMOGLOBIN ASSAY
Normal, healthy person 5.5–8.8% of total hemoglobin *or*
SI 0.05–0.08 (fraction of total hemoglobin)
Diabetic under control 7.5–11.4% of total hemoglobin
  Hemoglobin A_{1a} 1.8% of total hemoglobin
  Hemoglobin A_{1b} 0.8% of total hemoglobin
  Hemoglobin A_{1c} 3.56% of total hemoglobin

Purpose of the Test

Glycosylated hemoglobin refers to hemoglobin that has hooked up with glucose. The major glycosylated hemoglobin is hemoglobin A_{1c}, which is approximately 4 to 6% of the total hemoglobin. The other glycosylated hemoglobins are phosphoxylated glucose (A_{1a}) and phosphoxylated fructose (A_{1b}). Usually, a laboratory will report the total glycosylated hemoglobin level (hemoglobin A_1).

The reaction between glucose and hemoglobin is based on the blood glucose concentration. The higher the glucose concentration, the higher percentage of glycosylated hemoglobin. Since the reaction is not reversible, once the glucose adheres to the hemoglobin it remains glycosylated. Since the life span of a red blood cell is normally 120 days, measuring the glycosylated hemoglobin can assist in diabetic control assessment. It is not affected by recent changes in diet or medication, like fasting blood glucose, so the physician can determine diabetic control over a period of weeks or months. Diabetics who are poorly controlled will have a glycosylated hemoglobin value that is more than 12% of the total hemoglobin value.

Procedure

Venipuncture is performed to obtain 5 ml of blood in a test tube containing an anticoagulant (lavender-topped tube with EDTA or a green-topped tube with heparin).

Findings

Increase

Poorly controlled diabetes mellitus
Hyperglycemia

Interfering Factors

Anemia
Chronic renal failure
Clotting of specimen
Fetal-maternal transfusion
Hemodialysis
Hemorrhage
Hemolytic disease
Phlebotomies
Thalassemias

Nursing Implementation

The actions of the nurse resemble those used in other venipuncture procedures.

H

N O R M A L   V A L U E S

Hepatitis A antibody (Anti-HAV): negative
  IgM type: negative
  IgG type: negative
Hepatitis B core antibody (Anti-HBc): negative
  IgM type: negative
  IgG type: negative
Hepatitis Be antibody (Anti-HBe): negative
Hepatitis Be antigen (HbeAg): negative
Hepatitis B surface antibody (HBsAb): negative
Hepatitis B surface antigen (HBsAg): negative
Hepatitis C antibody (Anti-HCV): negative
Hepatitis Delta antibody (Anti-HDV): negative
  IgM type: negative
  IgG type: negative

Purpose of the Tests

Hepatitis A antibody test identifies the hepatitis A virus as the cause of infection. The specific antibody type distinguishes between current and past infection.

Hepatitis B core antibody test is used to assess the stage of hepatitis B infection.

Hepatitis Be antibody test helps to stage the course of the illness and is an indicator of prognosis for the infection.

Hepatitis Be antigen test is used in the diagnosis and prognosis of hepatitis B infection.

Hepatitis B surface antibody test is used to evaluate possible immunity or the need for vaccination in those people who are at high risk to develop hepatitis B infection. It is also used to evaluate the need for treatment after a "needlestick" incident.

Hepatitis B surface antigen test is used to identify the specific type of hepatitis and the acute or chronic stage of the infection.

glucocorticoids, glucose administered intravenously, hypoglycemic agents, insulin, lithium, phenothiazines, phenytoin)

Nursing Implementation

- *Pretest*

Instruct the patient to eat normally before the test.

- *During the Test*

The patient ingests a meal containing at least 100 g of carbohydrate.

Instruct the patient not to eat or drink for 2 hours after the meal is ingested.

Venipuncture is performed to obtain a blood glucose level 2 hours after the meal.

- *Posttest*

The patient resumes a normal diet.

HUMAN CHORIONIC GONADOTROPIN (hCG) • SERUM, URINE

NORMAL VALUES

SERUM

Male; nonpregnant female: Negative <3 mU/ml *or* SI <3 UL
Pregnant female
1 week gestation: 5–50 mU/ml *or* SI 5050 UL
4 weeks gestation: 1000–30,000 mU/ml *or* SI 1000–30,000 UL
6–8 weeks gestation: 12,000–270,000 mU/ml *or* SI 12,000–270,000 UL
12 weeks gestation: 15,000–270,000 mU/ml *or* SI 15,000–270,000 UL

URINE

Male; nonpregnant female: Negative
Pregnant female: Positive

Purpose of the Tests

Serum

This test is used to detect an early pregnancy, help confirm the diagnosis of a trophoblastic disorder, and monitor the postsurgical patient regarding the need for additional treatment.

Urine

This test confirms pregnancy within 6 days of conception. The test is also used to screen for an unknown pregnancy when a teratogenic medication or treatment must be given.

Procedure

Serum

A red-topped tube is used to obtain 7 ml of venous blood.

> ✓ QUALITY CONTROL
> To prevent hemolysis, venipuncture technique must be smooth, with a blood flow that fills the vacuum tube readily.

Urine

A clean plastic container is used to collect a first-voided morning specimen of urine.

Findings

Increase	*Decrease*
Pregnancy	Ectopic pregnancy
Hydatidiform mole	Threatened abortion
Choriocarcinoma	
Cancer (pancreas, lung, stomach, liver, colon, ovary, testis)	
Melanoma	
Multiple myeloma	

Interfering Factors

Serum

Recent radioactive isotope scan
Hemolysis

Urine

Hematuria
Bacteruria

Proteinuria
Detergent or soap in the container

Nursing Implementation

- *Pretest*

Serum

Schedule this test before or at least 7 days after a nuclear scan.

Urine

Instruct the patient to collect a single specimen in the laboratory collection container.

- *Posttest*

Urine

Ensure that the lid is in place and that the container label has the correct identification

Serum and Urine

On the requisition slip, include the date of the patient's last menstrual period.

Arrange for prompt delivery of the specimen to the laboratory.

✓ QUALITY CONTROL
If there is a delay before the analysis is performed, the laboratory must freeze the serum or refrigerate the urine.

HUMAN IMMUNODEFICIENCY VIRUS (HIV) TESTS • SERUM

NORMAL VALUES

ELISA assay: No HIV antibodies detected
Western blot: No HIV antibodies detected
Polymerase chain reaction (PCR) viral genome: No HIV antigen detected
CD4/CD8 (T4 helper/T8 suppressor) ratio: 0.5–3.3
C4 (T helper lymphocytes): 436–1394 cells/μL *or* SI 436–1394 × 10^6 cells/L

Purpose of the Tests

The ELISA test is used to screen for HIV infection and to screen blood donated for transfusion purposes. The Western blot test is used to confirm a positive ELISA test result. The PCR detects the HIV antigen at an early stage of infection. The CD4/CD8 ratio monitors progression of the disease and the C4 count evaluates the need to begin azathioprine (AZT) treatment.

Procedure

For each test, a red-topped tube is used to collect 7 ml of venous blood.

> ✓ QUALITY CONTROL
> The tourniquet should be tied lightly for a brief time to prevent pooling of cells in the vein at the site of blood collection. To prevent hemolysis, venipuncture technique must be smooth, with a blood flow that fills the vacuum tube readily.

Findings

Positive

Antigen tests: HIV infection
Antibody tests: HIV infection

Decrease

CD4:CD8 ratio: A value of <1 indicates AIDS.
CD4: A cell count of <300 cells/μL *or* SI <300 $\times$ 10^6 cells/L is an indicator for AZT treatment.

Interfering Factors

Hemolysis

Nursing Implementation

- *Pretest*

Because of confidentiality laws, an informed consent is often required before the test can be performed.

- *Posttest*

A positive ELISA antibody screen requires repeat testing by a Western blot or alternate antibody test. For the patient with a positive blood test:

1. Inform the patient that he or she cannot donate blood.

2. Explain that safe sex practices or abstaining from sexual intercourse helps prevent transmission of the disease.
3. Instruct that intravenous needles must not be shared.
4. Instruct the patient to continue with regular periodic examinations and follow-up laboratory testing. The pregnant female patient should inform her doctor of the positive test result because the virus can be transmitted from the infected mother to the fetus.

HUMAN LEUKOCYTE ANTIGEN (HLA TYPING)
• BLOOD

NORMAL VALUES

Specific leukocyte antigens are identified.

Purpose of the Test

In organ or bone marrow transplantation, HLA tissue typing is used to determine tissue compatibility between the donor and the recipient. With genetic compatibility between the donor and recipient, there is lower risk of rejection or graft-versus-host disease following transplant surgery. This test is also used to exclude paternity.

Procedure

Donor

A green-topped tube is filled with 7 to 10 ml of venous blood.

Recipient

A red-topped tube is used to obtain 7 to 10 ml of venous blood.

Findings

Incompatibility of donor and recipient tissues

Interfering Factors

Recent blood transfusion
Inadequate lymphocytes in the specimen

Nursing Implementation

- *Pretest*

Schedule this test before or 72 hours after any blood transfusion.

- *Posttest*

Arrange for prompt transport of the specimen to the laboratory. The analysis must be performed immediately on a fresh blood sample.

✓ QUALITY CONTROL
A prolonged delay or refrigeration of the specimen will yield an insufficient number of lymphocytes for the test.

17-HYDROXYCORTICOSTEROIDS • URINE

Synonym: 17-OHCS

NORMAL VALUES

Adult male: 4.5–12 mg/24 hours *or* SI 12.4–33.1 µmol/24 hours
Adult female: 2.5–10 mg/24 hours *or* SI 6.9–27.6 µmol/24 hours
Children
  8–12 years: <4.5 mg/24 hours *or* SI <12.4 µmol/24 hours
  <8 years: <1.5 mg/24 hours *or* SI <4.14 µmol/24 hours

Purpose of the Test

17-OHCS are urinary steroids (cortisol and cortisone metabolites) used to assess adrenal function. An increase in 17-OHCS in the urine reflects an increase in plasma cortisol. With the direct measurement of plasma cortisol and free cortisol, the frequency of 17-OHCS determinations has significantly decreased.

When assessing 17-OHCS values, it is necessary to consider the patient's body type. Obese or muscular individuals will have higher 17-OHCS levels than will those with normal body types because of an increase in cortisol metabolism. To adjust to body type, some clinicians correlate the 17-OHCS to the creatinine clearance.

Procedure

A 24-hour urine specimen is obtained. The urine is assessed by colorimetric reaction.

Findings

Increase	*Decrease*
Adrenal cancer	Addison's disease
Cushing's syndrome	Hypothyroidism
Extreme stress	Starvation liver failure
Hyperthyroidism	Renal failure
Pituitary tumor	Pregnancy

Interfering Factors

Failure to collect all the urine during the 24-hour collection period

Failure to keep specimen on ice or refrigerated

Medications (chloral hydrate, chlorpromazine, colchicine, erythromycin, estrogens, oral contraceptives, paraldehyde, quinidine, quinine, reserpine, spironolactone)

Nursing Implementation

* *Pretest*

Take the patient's medication history to assess for interfering factors.

Explain collection procedure to the patient, especially the need to collect *all* the urine for 24 hours.

Instruct the patient to avoid excessive physical activity during the testing period

* *During the Test*

At the start of the test, instruct the patient to void at 8 a.m. and discard this urine. The collection period begins at this time and all the urine is collected for 24 hours, including the 8 a.m. specimen of the following morning.

On the requisition slip and specimen label, write the patient's name and the time and date of the start and finish of the test period.

Keep the urine and collection container refrigerated or on ice during the collection period.

* *Posttest*

Arrange for prompt transport of the cooled specimen to the laboratory.

5-HYDROXYINDOLEACETIC ACID (5-HIAA)

• URINE

N O R M A L   V A L U E S

Adult: 1–9 mg/24 hours *or* SI 5–48 µmol/24 hours

Purpose of the Test

5-Hydroxyindoleacetic acid (5-HIAA) is a urinary metabolite of serotonin. The parent hormone, serotonin, and this urinary metabolite are produced by most carcinoid tumors. Because the elevated urine value serves as a marker for malignancy, this test is used to diagnose carcinoid tumors and provide ongoing evaluation of the stability of the tumor mass.

Procedure

For a 24-hour period, all urine is collected in a large container.

Findings

Increase

Carcinoid tumor (stomach, small intestine, colon, rectum, pancreas, bronchus, ovaries)
Celiac disease
Cystic fibrosis
Chronic intestinal obstruction

Decrease

Mental depression
Small bowel resection
Mastocytosis
Phenylketonuria

Interfering Factors

Numerous foods that contain serotonin
Numerous medications that react with the laboratory reagent

Nursing Implementation

• *Pretest*

Instruct the patient to avoid all foods that are high in serotonin for 48 hours before the test. These foods falsely elevate the test results and include avocados, tomatoes, bananas, plums, walnuts, pineapples, and eggplant.

For 48 hours before the test, discontinue all medications that interfere with the analysis procedure because they falsely elevate the results.

✓ QUALITY CONTROL

The specific medications to be eliminated depend on the method of laboratory analysis. To identify these medications, the nurse should call the laboratory beforehand.

• *During the Test*

For the 24-hour period of urine collection, the container is kept on ice or in the refrigerator.

• *Posttest*

Arrange for transport of the cooled specimen immediately.

Monotest: negative, nonreactive
Heterophil titer: <1:56
Epstein-Barr viral serology
  Viral capsid antigen (VCA) IgM: <1:10
  VCA-IgG: <1:10
  Epstein-Barr nuclear antigen (EBNA): <1:5
  Early antigen (EA): <1:10

Purpose of the Tests

These serologic tests are used to diagnose infectious mononucleosis. When the monotest and heterophil titer screening tests are negative, serology tests for the Epstein-Barr virus may be used. The VCA IgM and VCA IgG rise in the acute phase of illness and the EBNA and EA are increased in convalescence.

Procedure

A red-topped tube is used to collect 5 to 10 ml of venous blood.

Findings

Increase

Monotest and Heterophil Antibody tests: Infectious mononucleosis

Epstein-Barr Viral Serology: Infectious mononucleosis, nasopharyngeal cancer, Burkitt's lymphoma, Hodgkin's disease

Interfering Factors

None

Nursing Implementation

- *Pretest*

Schedule these tests to be performed at the onset of illness and again after 2 to 3 weeks. This provides data during the periods of acute and convalescent phases of illness.

- *Posttest*

On the requisition slip, write the date of the onset of illness.

INSULIN • SERUM OR PLASMA

N O R M A L   V A L U E S

FASTING
Adult: 5–25 µU/ml *or* SI 34–172 pmol/L
Newborn: 3–20 µU/ml *or* SI 21–138 pmol/L
1 hour after eating: 50–130 µU/ml *or* SI 347.3–902.8 pmol/L
2 hours after eating: <30 µU/ml *or* SI <208.4 pmol/L

Purpose of the Test

Insulin levels are determined to assess for insulin-producing tumors, confirm suspected insulin-resistant states, and as part of the evaluation of glucocorticoid insufficiency.

Procedure

Insulin levels may be assessed by random venous sampling or during a glucose tolerance test. A specimen is obtained by venipuncture and collected in an anticoagulated tube. The specimen is assessed by RIA.

Findings

Increase	*Decrease*
Acromegaly	IDDM
Cushing's syndrome	Hypopituitarism
Hyperinsulinism	
Insulinoma	
Liver disease	
Pancreatic lesions	
Vagal stimulation	

Interfering Factors

Noncompliance with test protocol
Insulin antibodies
Medications (ACTH, catecholamines, colchicine, diazoxide, oral contraceptives, phenytoin, steroids, sulfonylureas, thyroid hormones, vinblastine)

Nursing Implementation

Care varies according to whether a fasting sample is used or the insulin level is being obtained as part of the GTT (see pp. 168–170 for this test).

• Pretest

Take a medication history to determine if any interfering drugs are being taken. Check to determine if these drugs are to be withheld. If the patient is receiving insulin therapy, the insulin is withheld until the test is performed.

Assess the patient's stress level, which may increase endogenous glucocorticoid secretion.

If a fasting insulin sample is to be drawn, instruct the patient not to eat or drink for 7 hours before the blood is drawn.

• During the Test

Observe the patient for hyperglycemia if the insulin is withheld and for hypoglycemia because of the fasting state.

If performed with a GTT, a blood sample for insulin is obtained each time a glucose level specimen is drawn.

✓ QUALITY CONTROL
Send the specimen to the laboratory immediately, as it must be centrifuged within 30 minutes and frozen until the assay can be performed.

• Posttest

The patient resumes normal medication schedule and diet therapies.

INTRAVENOUS PYELOGRAM • RADIOGRAPHY

Synonyms: IVP, excretory urogram, EUG, intravenous urography, IVU, IUG

NORMAL VALUES

Normal renal tissue is present, with no indication of inflammation, fibrosis, necrosis, or tumor cells.

Purpose of the Test

The intravenous pyelogram is a basic urologic procedure that uses contrast medium and radiography to visualize the anatomy and function of the urinary tract. The intravenous pyelogram is used to evaluate the structure and function of the kidneys, ureters, and bladder. It assesses the cause of nontraumatic hematuria, locates the precise site of obstruction, and investigates the cause of flank pain or renal colic.

Procedure

An initial x-ray film is taken to provide baseline information. After an intravenous injection of contrast material, timed radiographs are taken of the urinary tract. Films at 1 minute visualize the kidneys; at 3 to 5 minutes, the renal collecting system is visualized; at 10 minutes, the ureters are seen; and at 20 to 30 minutes filling of the bladder is seen. A postvoiding film demonstrates the ability of the bladder to empty. The test requires 1 to 1½ hours to complete.

Findings

Hydronephrosis
Renal or ureteral calculi
Hydroureter
Polycystic kidney disease
Tumor
Pyelonephritis
Renal tuberculosis
Absent kidney
Congenital anomalies
Nonfunctioning kidney

Interfering Factors

Renal failure
Feces, gas, or barium in the colon
Recent gallbladder series
Failure to maintain a nothing-by-mouth status

Nursing Implementation

- *Pretest*

Ask the patient about any history of allergy to shellfish or iodine or a previous reaction to an x-ray study that used contrast medium.

Schedule the intravenous pyelogram before any barium test or
gallbladder series that also used iodinated contrast material.

Explain the procedure to the patient and obtain a written consent from the patient or person legally designated to make
health care decisions for the patient.

Instruct the patient regarding the pretest bowel cleansing procedure that removes gas and fecal matter. This includes taking the prescribed laxative or cathartic the night before the
test and an enema or suppository on the morning of the
test.

Instruct the patient to discontinue food intake for 8 hours before the test. Fluids are permitted.

> ✓ QUALITY CONTROL
> Patients who are dehydrated are at high risk for the develop-
> ment of renal failure as a result of the toxic effect of the con-
> trast medium on the kidney tissues. Adequate hydration before
> and after the test is essential.

Ensure that recent blood urea nitrogen and creatinine test results are posted in the chart. These tests help identify patients who are at risk and help determine a safe dose of contrast medium.

Record baseline vital signs.

- *During the Test*

Assist the patient as the contrast medium is administered. It is
common for the patient to experience a brief burning sensation
or a metallic taste, or both.

✪ **COMPLICATION ALERT** ✪ During the test, a small number of patients have a vasovagal response to the contrast material. Observe the patient for flushing, hypotension, and bradycardia. Intravenous epinephrine and oxygen should be on hand. An emergency cart is maintained in the radiology suite at all times.

• *Posttest*

Take the vital signs and record the results.

Continue the intravenous fluid replacement and encourage the patient to take oral fluids.

Observe for complication of allergy to the contrast medium and nephrotoxicity. Impaired renal function can occur from 1 to 4 days after the study is completed. Most times it is a transitory problem and the kidneys return to their baseline level of function.

IRON STUDIES • **SERUM**

N O R M A L   V A L U E S

Serum iron (Fe)
  Adult male: 65–175 µg/dl or SI 11.6–31.3 µmol/L
  Adult female: 50–170 µg/dl or SI 9–30.4 µmol/L
Transferrin (Tf)
  Adult 16–60 years: 200–400 mg/dl or SI 2–4 g/L
Total iron-binding capacity (TBIC): 218–385 (g/dl or SI 39–69 µmol/L
Transferrin saturate: 20–50%
Ferritin
  Adult male: 20–250 ng/ml or SI 20–250 µg/L
  Adult female: 10–120 ng/ml or SI 10–120 µg/L

Purpose of the Tests

These tests provide an estimate of total iron storage and information regarding the nutritional status of the individual. They help distinguish between iron deficiency anemia and the anemia of chronic disease. They also confirm the presence of iron overload and hematochromatosis.

Procedure

A red-topped tube is used to collect 7 ml of venous blood. This blood sample is drawn before other blood samples that require vacuum tubes with anticoagulant.

> ✓ QUALITY CONTROL
> The tourniquet is applied loosely and is not kept in place for long. To prevent hemolysis, the venipuncture must be smooth, with a blood flow that fills the vacuum tube readily.

Findings

Increase

Iron:
Anemias (pernicious, aplastic, hemolytic, thalassemia)
Hemochromatosis
Excess iron replacement
Poisoning (iron, lead)
Acute leukemia
Acute hepatitis
Transferrin:
Iron deficiency anemia
TIBC:
Anemias (iron deficiency, hypochromic)
Transferrin saturation:
Iron toxicity
Hemochromatosis
Thalassemia
Nephrosis
Hepatitis
Ferritin:
Hemochromatosis
Iron overload
Acute leukemia
Liver
Inflammatory or infectious disease

Decrease

Iron:
Iron deficiency anemia
Infection (acute or chronic)
Malignancy
Starvation
Transferrin:
Inflammation
Necrosis
Malignancy
Malnutrition
Liver disease
Nephrotic syndrome
TIBC:
Anemias (pernicious, aplastic, hemolytic, thalassemia)
Hemochromatosis
Malignancy
Renal disease
Transferrin saturation:
Iron deficiency anemia
Chronic infection
Malignancy
Ferritin:
Iron deficiency anemia

Interfering Factors

Recent administration of radioisotopes (ferritin)
Hemolysis (serum iron, iron saturation)
Lipemia (transferrin)
Recent blood transfusion (serum iron)

Nursing Implementation

- *Pretest*

Schedule these laboratory tests in the morning hours and
(a) before or a few days after a blood transfusion, (b) before any nuclear scans.

Instruct the patient to fast from food and fluid for 8 hours before the tests for transferrin levels. If the patient takes an iron supplement, include this information on the requisition slip.

- *Posttest*

Arrange for prompt transport of the specimen to the laboratory.

> ✓ QUALITY CONTROL
> The cells must be separated from the serum without delay. Hemolysis causes a false elevation.

KETONES • SERUM, URINE

Synonyms: Acetoacetate, acetones

NORMAL VALUES

SERUM
Negative: <1 mg/dl *or* SI <0.1 nmol/L

URINE
No ketones

Purpose of the Test

Without adequate insulin, three major ketone bodies accumulate in the blood and are excreted in the urine. These ketone bodies are acetone, acetoacetic acid, and beta-hydroxybutyric acid. Ketones form as fats and fatty acids are broken down.

Serum ketone levels are measured to distinguish between diabetic ketoacidosis and hyperosmolar coma. With diabetic ketoacidosis, incomplete fatty acid metabolism leads to increasing ketones in the blood. Patients with hyperosmolar coma produce minimal or no ketosis in the presence of extremely high levels of serum glucose. The mechanism of maintaining nearly normal ketone levels in hyperosmolar coma is not known. It is theorized that these patients have sufficient insulin to break down fatty acids or are glucagon-resistant.

Urine is tested for ketone bodies to evaluate the patient with diabetes mellitus and to diagnose carbohydrate deprivation. The concentration of urine ketones can be used to adjust insulin requirements in the diabetic and to monitor patients on low-carbohydrate diets.

Procedure

Serum

Venipuncture is performed to obtain 1 ml of blood in a red-topped tube.

Urine

There are a variety of commercial products available for testing ketones in the urine; such as, Acetest tablet, Ketostix, and Keto-Diastix. With the Acetest tablet, one drop of urine is dropped on a tablet. With the sticks, the paper strip is dipped in fresh urine. The color change of the tablet or on the strip is compared to the chart provided by the manufacturer to determine the presence and concentration of ketones.

Findings

Increase

Alcoholic ketoacidosis
Decreased caloric intake
Eclampsia
Isopropanol poisoning
Propranolol poisoning
Starvation
Uncontrolled diabetes mellitus
Gierke disease

Nursing Implementation

Serum

The nurse's duties are similar to those performed in other venipuncture procedures.

- *Pretest*

Urine

Instruct the patient about the double-void technique.

- *During the Test*

Urine

Instruct the patient to void, discard this urine, wait 30 minutes and void into a clean, dry container.
Check voided urine within 60 minutes.
Method of checking for ketones varies with the product. Follow manufacturer's guidelines.

- *Posttest*

Urine

Document the results, usually on a flow chart.
Adjust insulin dosage as ordered based on the results.

L

• VENOUS

Synonym: Lactate

NORMAL VALUES

1–2 mEq/L *or* SI 1–2 µmol/L

Purpose of the Test

Lactate levels are used to support the diagnosis of cellular hypoxia. If the cells do not receive adequate oxygen, anaerobic metabolism will occur. Lactic acid is the by-product of anaerobic metabolism. Rising lactate levels indicate a need to examine O_2 transport and consumption parameters. High lactate levels (>4 mmol/L) indicate higher mortality rates.

Procedure

A venipuncture is performed to obtain 1 ml of blood which is placed in a gray-topped tube.

Findings

Increase	*Decrease*
Alcoholism	Hypothermia
Diabetic ketoacidosis	
Hyperthermia	
Liver failure	
Malignancies	
Peritonitis	
Shock states	

Interfering Factors

Noncompliance with dietary and activity restrictions
Medications (acetaminophen [large doses], ethanol [large dose], epinephrine, fructose, sorbitol)

Nursing Implementation

The nurse takes actions similar to those taken with other venipuncture procedures.

- *Pretest*

Assess possibility of alcohol ingestion within the previous 24 hours and report if taken.

Instruct the patient to lie quietly for 2 hours before the blood is drawn.

- *During the Test*

No tourniquet should be applied, and the patient should not clench their fist.

Send the specimen to the laboratory immediately.

- *Posttest*

Advise the patient to resume a normal diet and activity level.

LACTOSE TOLERANCE TEST • BLOOD, URINE, FECES

N O R M A L   V A L U E S

Adult
Blood glucose: 20–30 mg/dl *or* SI 1.1–1.7 µmol/L
Urine lactose (24-hour): 12–40 mg/dl *or* SI 0.7–2.2 µmol/L
Feces: pH 7–8; glucose <1+
Child
Urine lactose (24-hour): <1.5 mg/100 dl

Purpose of the Test

This test verifies lactose intolerance–lactase insufficiency. It is used in the workup for abdominal distention, chronic diarrhea, and abdominal cramps associated with the ingestion of milk. It is also used to investigate the cause of malabsorption syndrome.

Procedure

The fasting patient takes an oral dose of lactose with 200 to 300 ml of water. The usual dose is 50 g or 0.75 to 1.5 g/kg of body weight, but a smaller dose is used for children or for patients suspected of having severe disease. Diagnostic results are obtained from the analysis of serial blood samples, a 24-hour urine collection, or a sample of feces. In some cases, the blood test may be combined with either the urine test or the stool test.

Blood. Gray-topped (fluoride) tubes or capillary tubes are used to collect small venous samples (fasting, baseline specimen, and specimens at 30, 60, 120, 180, and 240 minutes).

Urine. After ingestion of the lactose, all urine specimens are collected in a glass container for 24 hours.

Feces. Five hours after ingestion of lactose, a stool sample is collected in a clean, dry container.

Findings

Increase

Lactose intolerance–lactase insufficiency
Crohn's disease
Ulcerative colitis
Small bowel resection giardiasis
Sprue
Cystic fibrosis
Bowel infection

Interfering Factors

Failure to maintain dietary and exercise restrictions
Delayed emptying of the stomach
Vomiting
Diabetes mellitus

Nursing Implementation

• *Pretest*

Instruct the patient that for 8 hours before and during the test, there can be no food intake, smoking, or gum chewing.

✓ QUALITY CONTROL
Changes in gastric motility and gastric emptying affect the rate of absorption and alter the test results.

• *During the Test*

Assess for any signs of watery diarrhea, abdominal cramps, or nausea.

Notify the physician of any vomiting, since this could affect the amount and rate of lactose absorption. Some laboratories require activity restriction during the test.

- *Posttest*

After 4 hours, when the blood work is completed, the patient can resume activity and diet.

Remind the patient to continue with collection of the urine for 24 hours and to collect a fecal specimen in the fifth hour of the test, as prescribed.

> ✓ QUALITY CONTROL
> Label every specimen with the date and time of the collection. The laboratory slip should indicate the time of lactose administration as well as the times of specimen collection.

LAPAROSCOPY (PERITONEOSCOPY) • ENDOSCOPY

N O R M A L   V A L U E S

No abnormalities of the ovaries, fallopian tubes, uterus, liver, or peritoneal cavity are noted.

Purpose of the Test

Laparoscopy is used to investigate the cause of abdominal or pelvic pain, detect endometriosis or an ectopic pregnancy, identify a pelvic or abdominal mass, investigate suspected liver disease or the cause of ascites, or determine if cancer is present or has metastasized. Preoperative cancer staging may be done.

- *Procedure*

After inflating the peritoneal cavity with carbon dioxide or nitrous oxide, the laparoscope is inserted through one or two small abdominal incisions. It provides visualization of the peritoneal cavity and the organs within, including the uterus, ovaries, fallopian tubes, liver, gallbladder, and peritoneum. Biopsy of abnormal tissue and/or aspiration of a sample of ascites fluid may be performed.

Findings

Ovarian cyst
Endometriosis
Ectopic pregnancy
Uterine fibroid tumors
Abscess
Pelvic inflammatory disease
Adhesions
Abnormality of the fallopian tubes
Malignancy
Cirrhosis of the liver

Interfering Factors

Failure to maintain a nothing-by-mouth status
Obesity
Adhesions
Advanced abdominal wall malignancy
Hernia
Severe cardiorespiratory disease
Intestinal obstruction
Uncooperative patient

Nursing Implementation

• *Pretest*

Provide information regarding skin preparation and bathing,
taking preventive antibiotics, and a review of post procedure
instructions that includes care of the incision, activity and exercise, and pain control.
Instruct the patient to discontinue all food and fluids for
8 hours before the procedure is performed.
Obtain written consent.
Ensure that all preoperative laboratory work is completed and
that the results are in the chart.
Assess and record the vital signs.
Premedicate with prescribed narcotic-analgesics such as midalo-
zam (Versed) and meperidine (Demerol).
Position the patient on the laparoscopy tilt table, applying
straps over the chest and thighs.

- *During the Test*

Insert the indwelling catheter into the bladder and connect it
to the urinary collection system.

Apply electronic monitoring devices for vital signs, ECG, and
oxygen saturation.

If a biopsy specimen is obtained, place the tissue in a glass container with preservative. Identify the tissue source on the
container and the requisition slip. Ascites fluid is placed in
a sterile collection container and also is labeled appropriately.

✓ QUALITY CONTROL

On completion of the procedure, the laparoscope must be disassembled, thoroughly cleaned, and disinfected. Since the instrument is reused, these measures prevent transmission of infection.

- *Posttest*

Monitor the vital signs every 30 minutes for 4 hours or until
stable.

Ensure that the dressing remains dry and intact.

Monitor for voiding and urinary output.

Once the patient is alert, encourage ambulation and the oral
intake of fluids. A light diet begins in about 6 hours. Car-
bonated beverages are avoided for 24 to 36 hours.

Provide pain medication as needed. Advise the patient that the
instilled gas can cause some pain in the abdomen and shoulder for 24 to 36 hours, until the gas is absorbed and exhaled.

Instruct the patient to restrict physical activity for a few days
until the incisions are healed. Sutures are removed in
10 days.

Ensure that a family member is aware of the plan of care and
is able to help the patient at home, as needed.

✪ **COMPLICATION ALERT** ✪ Because of the potential
for bleeding, the nurse assesses for bloody drainage from the incision and signs of shock (hypotension and tachycardia). Infection
can also occur, so the patient is monitored for fever, sweating,
tachycardia, and abdominal pain.

LEUKOCYTE ALKALINE PHOSPHATASE (LAP) • PERIPHERAL BLOOD

NORMAL VALUES

11–95 (Jacobs, et al., 1996)

Purpose of the Test

This test helps differentiate chronic myelogenous leukemia from leukemoid reaction and other myeloproliferative diseases. It is also useful in the evaluation of Hodgkin's disease and its response to therapy.

Procedure

Fingerstick or earlobe puncture is used to make six slides with smears of the peripheral blood. As an alternative, a green-topped tube with heparin or oxalate anticoagulant is used to collect 7 ml of venous blood.

Findings

Increase	*Decrease*
Leukemoid reactions	Chronic myelogenous leukemia
Hodgkin's disease	
Acute lymphoblastic leukemia	Acute monocytic leukemia
Hairy cell leukemia	Acute myeloid leukemia
Polycythemia vera	Congestive heart failure
Myelofibrosis	Cirrhosis
	Collagen disease

• Interfering Factors

Pregnancy
Acute stress
Neutropenia
Delay in the final preparation of slides

Nursing Implementation

• Pretest

To ensure a valid test, verify that the recent peripheral blood neutrophil count is greater than 1000/mm^3.

• *Posttest*

Arrange for immediate transport of the slides or blood specimen to the laboratory.

✓ QUALITY CONTROL
To avoid rejection of the specimen, the slides must be fixed in preservative within 30 minutes.

LIPASE • SERUM

NORMAL VALUES
Adult: <200 U/L

Purpose of the Test

This test is used to diagnose pancreatitis and pancreatic disease.

Procedure

Venipuncture is performed to obtain 5 to 10 ml of blood in a red-topped tube.

✓ QUALITY CONTROL
To prevent hemolysis, venipuncture must be smooth, with a blood flow that fills the vacutainer readily.

Findings

Increase

Acute pancreatitis
Pancreatic cyst or pseudocyst
Obstruction of pancreatic duct
Gallstone
Primary biliary cirrhosis

Interfering Factors

Heparin
Narcotics
Hemolysis
Failure to maintain the NPO status

Nursing Implementation

• *Pretest*

In dialysis patients, insure that the lipase blood sample is obtained prior to a dialysis treatment. The heparin used during dialysis would cause a false rise in the lipase value.

Instruct the patient to discontinue all food and fluid for 12 hours before the test.

LIPIDS • SERUM

Synonym: Lipoprotein-cholesterol fractionation

N O R M A L   V A L U E S

Lipids, total: 400–800 mg/dl *or* SI 4.0–8.0 g/L
Cholesterol, total: 120–200 mg/dl *or* SI 3.11–5.18 µmol/L
Low-density lipoprotein (LDL): <130 mg/dl *or* SI <3.37 µmol/L
High-density lipoprotein (HDL)
Male: 44–45 mg/dl *or* SI 1.24–1.27 µmol/L
Female: 55 mg/dl *or* SI 1.425 µmol/L
LDL:HDL ratio: <3
Triglycerides
Male: <40 years 46–316 mg/dl *or* SI 0.52–3.57 µmol/L
>50 years 75–313 mg/dl *or* SI 0.85–3.5 µmol/L
Female: <40 years 37–174 mg/dl *or* SI 0.42–1.97 µmol/L
>50 years 52–200 mg/dl *or* SI 0.59–2.26 µmol/L

Purpose of the Test

Lipid levels are used to identify individuals at risk for CAD and as an evaluation tool to determine the effectiveness of "heart-healthy" changes in lifestyle.

Most lipids are bound to protein in the blood and are called lipoproteins. In the laboratory, lipoproteins are separated by electrophoresis. Fractionation of the lipoproteins is then performed according to their density. The following groups have been identified: very low-density lipoproteins (VLDL), which are made up of 70% triglycerides; low-density lipoproteins (LDL), which are made up of 45% cholesterol; and high-density lipoproteins (HDL).

There is a high correlation between elevated VLDL and LDL with CAD. Research has shown that HDL may protect from CAD, since it seems to inhibit the uptake of LDL.

Procedure

A venipuncture is necessary for a lipid profile. Two red-topped tubes of 7-ml capacity are required. If a cholesterol level determination is performed as a screening test, a drop or two of blood is obtained from a fingerstick using a sterile lancet, and the blood is collected in a capillary pipette.

Findings

Increase in Cholesterol

Alcoholism
Arteriosclerosis
CAD
Diabetes mellitus
Hepatitis (early stage)
High-fat diet
Myxedema
Obstructed bile duct
Pancreatitis

Decrease in Cholesterol

Hyperalimentation
Hyperthyroidism
Liver disease
Malabsorption
Malnutrition

Increase in HDL

Alcoholism
Diabetes mellitus
Exercise
Myxedema
Nephrotic syndrome
Pancreatitis

Decrease in HDL

Arteriosclerosis
Hyperalimentation
Hypothyroidism
Malabsorption
Malnutrition

Increase in LDL

Alcoholism
CAD
Diabetes mellitus
Nephrotic syndrome
Pancreatitis

Decrease in LDL

Arteriosclerosis
Hyperalimentation
Malabsorption
Malnutrition

Increase in Triglycerides	*Decrease in Triglycerides*
Alcoholism	Hyperalimentation
Arteriosclerosis	Malabsorption
Diabetes mellitus	Malnutrition
Myxedema	
Nephrotic syndrome	
Pancreatitis	

Interfering Factors

Diet high in fat
Dieting
Trauma
Infarction
Medications (estrogens, steroids, birth control pills, antihyper-
lipidemia)

Nursing Implementation

The nursing actions are similar to those of other venipunctures.
In addition, review the following.

- *Pretest*

Ask patient if they have maintained a normal diet for the previous 2 to 3 weeks.

Instruct the patient to fast for 10 to 12 hours before the blood
sample is taken. If only a cholesterol screening is planned,
instruct the patient to refrain from eating a high-fat diet for
12 hours before the blood is drawn.

- *Posttest*

Review results with the patient. If the patient is at risk for CAD,
diet and exercise education may be necessary.

LIVER BIOPSY • PATHOLOGY

NORMAL VALUE

The liver cells are normal, with no evidence of inflammation,
scarring, degeneration, or tumor.

Purpose of the Test

Liver biopsy is done when there is unexplained enlargement of the liver, abnormal liver function tests, and jaundice. The biopsy is used to diagnose the liver pathology and to help evaluate the extent of the disease process.

Procedure

The liver biopsy is done by percutaneous needle aspiration that removes a small sample of liver tissue.

The needle is placed between the anterior and midaxillary lines, usually in the sixth or seventh intercostal space. While the patient holds his or her breath on expiration, the needle is inserted quickly and a 10 ml syringe is used to aspirate the tissue. Once the needle is removed, the patient resumes breathing.

Findings

Cirrhosis
Sarcoidosis
Chronic hepatitis B
Cyst
Cancer (primary or metastatic)

Interfering Factors

Obesity
Infection in right pleural cavity or right upper quadrant of the
    abdomen
Noncooperative behavior
Abnormal clotting ability

Nursing Implementation

- *Pretest*

Obtain a signed consent.
Provide teaching about the procedure, the positioning and
    breathing instructions, and the posttest instructions. To alle-
    viate anxiety, provide reassurance and support as needed.
Instruct the patient to discontinue all food and fluids for
    8 hours before the test.
Check that a recent PT, PTT, and platelet count have been

done and that the results are within safety guidelines for this procedure. The laboratory reports are placed in the chart and the physician is notified of abnormal values.

> ✓ QUALITY CONTROL
> Patients with liver disorders may also have poor clotting ability. The prothrombin time should not be more that 3 seconds above the control time, and the platelet count should be >100,000 mm.

Take baseline vital signs and record them in the patient's chart.

Administer any prescribed pretest medication about one hour before the test. Meperidine (Demerol) or diazepam (Valium) are commonly used for analgesia and relaxation.

Position the patient on his or her left side or in supine position, with the arm under the head. The skin is cleansed with antiseptic and draped with a sterile cloth.

• During the Test

Stand beside the patient to provide reassurance and to help maintain immobility.

Assist with the placement of the tissue into the specimen jar that contains formalin or saline.

Label the specimen with the patient's data and the source of the tissue.

Cover the aspiration site with a sterile dressing, take vital signs, and position the patient on the right side.

Record the procedure and assessment data in the patient's chart.

• Posttest

To promote clotting, the patient remains positioned on the right side with a pillow pressing on the area for 1–2 hours.

Vital signs are taken every 15 minutes for one hour, every hour for 4 hours, and every 4 hours thereafter.

Assesses for signs of bleeding on a frequent or regular basis.

Abnormal signs include swelling of the abdomen, ecchymosis in the dependent area of skin over the rib cage, tachycardia, and hypotension.

The patient can resume food and fluid intake as desired. Bedrest remains in effect for 12 to 24 hours.

⊙ **COMPLICATION ALERT** ⊙ In addition to the assessment for bleeding (ecchymosis, pallor, diaphoresis), the nurse should also observe for signs of a pneumothorax (dyspnea, cyanosis, apprehension) and peritonitis (persistent severe abdominal or shoulder pain, fever, and a board-like, distended abdomen). Hypotension, tachycardia, and shock can occur in all of these complications.

LUNG BIOPSY, OPEN AND PERCUTANEOUS	• PATHOLOGY

Synonym: Fine needle biopsy of the lung

N O R M A L V A L U E S
Normal tissue

Purpose of the Test

A lung biopsy is performed to remove lung tissue so that the cells may be examined microscopically for pathologic features to diagnose pulmonary disorders such as cancer and sarcoidosis. Lung biopsy can confirm the diagnosis of fibrosis and degenerative or inflammatory diseases of the lung. A variety of methods are used to obtain these lung cells. Tissue samples may be obtained by bronchoscopy (see pp. 46–49), by fine needle biopsy, or by open biopsy. With an open biopsy, surgery is required, with its potential risks.

Procedure

For an open biopsy of the lung, a thoracotomy is required, which is a surgical procedure. After a small incision is made in the chest wall, the lung is exposed and tissue is excised. A chest tube or tubes are inserted to restore negative pleural pressure.

For a percutaneous needle biopsy, under the guidance of CT scanning or fluoroscopy, a biopsy needle is inserted through the chest wall into a lesion and a specimen is aspirated for histological examination.

Findings

Carcinomas
Granulomas
Infections
Sarcoidosis

Interfering Factors

Noncompliance with dietary restrictions
Smoking
Obesity

Nursing Implementation

Follow hospital protocol for the preoperative and postoperative care of a patient requiring a thoracotomy for an open-lung biopsy. For a percutaneous lung biopsy:

- *Pretest*

Assess the patient for bleeding disorders, as the needle path may be close to major vessels.
Instruct the patient about the procedure and the need to remain still and not cough when instructed not to move.
Assess the patient's history for contraindications to fine needle biopsy: pulmonary hypertension, severe chronic obstructive lung disease, or arteriovenous malformation.
Transport the patient to the CT laboratory; if fluoroscopy is planned, bring the patient to the radiology department.

- *During the Test*

The patient is positioned according to the location of the lesion.
The skin is marked as a guide for needle insertion.
Skin preparation is carried out, and the area is draped.
A local anesthetic is given.
The biopsy needle is inserted, and samples are taken.
A pathologist may be present to prepare slides from the aspirated specimen. If a pathologist is not present, send the specimen in fixative to the laboratory.

- *Posttest*

Observe the patient for a minimum of 2 hours.
A chest x-ray study is usually ordered 1 to 2 hours after the procedure to identify any pneumothoraces.

⊘ **COMPLICATION ALERT** ⊘ Both an open and a percutaneous lung biopsy can cause bleeding, pneumothorax, and infection. In addition, a percutaneous lung biopsy may cause a perforation leading to a bile leak.

LUNG SCANS	• RADIOGRAPHY

Synonyms: Ventilation scan, perfusion scan, ventilation-perfusion scan, V̇/Q̇ scan, ventilation-perfusion scintiphotography

N O R M A L   V A L U E S

Normal ventilation and perfusion
Ventilation-perfusion ratio of 0.85 or greater

Purpose of the Test

Ventilation studies may be performed to evaluate patients with decreased pulmonary function. There are two types of lung scans: a *ventilation scan* and a *perfusion scan*. Ventilation scans are performed to evaluate the distribution of gas within the lungs. The patient inhales a radioactive gas and a scanner records the distribution of the gas as it enters and leaves the lungs. Perfusion scans evaluate arterial pulmonary blood flow. A radioactive dye is given intravenously and a scintillation camera records the distribution of the dye as it passes through the right side of the heart into the pulmonary arterial bed.

Ventilation and perfusion scans (V̇/Q̇ scans) may be performed together so that they can be compared to identify mismatching of ventilation and perfusion. V̇/Q̇ scans are most often ordered to confirm the diagnosis of pulmonary emboli. Although pulmonary angiography is the most specific diagnostic tool for pulmonary emboli, it is invasive. A V̇/Q̇ scan is less invasive and therefore less dangerous.

Procedure

For a perfusion scan, serum albumin is tagged with a radioisotope and given intravenously. As the tagged albumin passes through the right side of the heart into the pulmonary artery, a radiation detector scan of the lungs shows the diffusion of the radioactive albumin throughout the pulmonary vessels.

With a ventilation scan, xenon-133, xenon-127, or krypton-81m is given via inhalation. Multiple scans are taken during (1) wash-in, as the radioactive gas builds up in the lung; (2) equilibrium, as the gas reaches its plateau within the lung; and (3) washout, as the radioactive gas is exhaled.

Findings

Pulmonary vascular occlusion resulting from thrombus, cysts, abscesses, carcinomas, necrotizing pneumonia.

Inadequate ventilation resulting from atelectasis, chronic obstructive pulmonary disease, adult respiratory distress syndrome, retained secretions, pleural effusion, pneumonia, pneumothorax.

Interfering Factors

Uncooperative patient

Nursing Implementation

• *Pretest*

Inform the patient about the procedure and ensure patient cooperation.

Explain to the patient that the ventilation scan must be performed in the nuclear medicine department. Some hospitals have portable perfusion scanners.

Advise the patient that with the ventilation scan the inhaled gas should be held in the lungs for 20 seconds when instructed to do so.

Schedule other radionuclide tests 24 to 48 hours after the perfusion scan.

• *During the Test*

Maintain the patient in an upright position for the ventilation scan. This position is maintained for at least 15 minutes.

If the patient is unable to maintain the upright position, a supine position may be used with the gamma camera underneath the patient.

After the radioactive gas is inhaled, encourage the patient to hold the breath for 20 seconds.

Radiolabeled albumin is given to the patient intravenously.

Six different views of the chest are obtained: anterior, posterior, right and left lateral, and right and left oblique.

LUPUS ERYTHEMATOSUS TEST • SERUM

Synonyms: LE prep, LE slide cell test, lupus test, lupus erythematosus cell test

N O R M A L   V A L U E S

Negative; no LE cells are present.

Purpose of the Test

The LE test is used to help diagnose lupus erythematosus and to monitor the response to treatment. In autoimmune disease, the serum contains antibodies that are directed against cell nuclei of one's own body tissues. In systemic lupus erythematosus, the antinuclear antibody is usually IgG and is called the *LE factor.* The antibody reacts with the deoxyribonucleoprotein of leukocytes by attaching to the nucleus and infiltrating it. After infiltration, the altered cell becomes a homogeneous mass of cytoplasm and is then called an *LE body.* Other neutrophils and phagocytes surround the LE body and engulf it by phagocytosis. After phagocytosis, the final cell, the *LE cell,* is a polymorphonuclear leukocyte with a lysed nucleus as an inclusion body. In systemic lupus erythematosus, the LE cells are found in the bone marrow and peripheral blood.

Procedure

A green-topped tube is used to collect 7 to 10 ml of venous blood.

Findings

Increase

Systemic lupus erythematosus
Rheumatoid arthritis
Chronic active hepatitis (lupoid hepatitis)
Scleroderma
Drug hypersensitivity
Drug-induced lupus syndrome

Interfering Factors

Severe leukopenia
Neutropenia
Heparin
Inadequate volume of blood sample

Nursing Implementation

- *Pretest*

If heparin has been administered, schedule the test 2 days after the heparin is discontinued.

On the laboratory requisition slip, list the medications taken by the patient.

- *Posttest*

Arrange for transport of the specimen to the laboratory within 30 minutes.

LUTEINIZING HORMONE (LH) • SERUM, URINE

N O R M A L   V A L U E S

SERUM
Adult
Male: 1–8 mU/ml *or* SI 1–8 U/L1–8 mU/ml *or* SI 1–8 U/L
Female
Follicular phase: 1–12 mU/ml *or* SI 1–12 U/L
Midcycle peak: 16–104 mU/ml *or* SI 16–104 U/L
Luteal phase: 1–12 mU/ml *or* SI 1–12 U/L
Postmenopausal: 16–66 mU/ml *or* SI 16–66 U/L
Child (6 months–10 years): 1–5 mU/ml *or* SI 1–5 U/L

URINE
Adult
Male: 9–23 U/24 hours
Female: 4–30 U/24 hours
Child
Male (1–10 years): <1–5.6 U/24 hours
Female (1–10 years): 1.4–4.9 U/24 hours

Purpose of the Test

This test helps diagnose the cause of gonadal dysfunction, including delayed sexual development, amenorrhea, and menstrual irregularity. It also is used as part of infertility evaluation.

Procedure

Serum

A red-topped or green-topped tube is used to collect 5 to 7 ml of venous blood.

Urine

A large bottle is used to collect urine for 24 hours. Some laboratories require the addition of boric, acetic, or hydrochloric acid. Other laboratories require no preservative in the bottle.

Findings

Increase

Primary gonadal dysfunction
Polycystic ovary syndrome
Postmenopause
Pituitary adenoma
Castration
Ovarian failure

Decrease

Malnutrition
Anorexia nervosa
Severe stress
Congenital adrenal hyperplasia
Adrenal tumor
Pituitary or hypothalamus disorder
Delayed puberty

Interfering Factors

Recent radioactive isotope scan

Nursing Implementation

• Pretest

Serum

Schedule this test before or at least 7 days after a nuclear scan.

✓ QUALITY CONTROL
The measurement of LH is carried out by radioimmunoassay. The radioisotopes of the scan would interfere with the analysis and results.

Urine

Provide both written and verbal instructions regarding the collection of urine.

- *During the Test*

Urine

The first-voided specimen of the morning is discarded and the urine collection period begins at 8 a.m.

All urine collected in the 24-hour period is placed in the container. This includes the first-voided specimen of the next morning.

Keep the specimen and container on ice or refrigerated during the collection period.

- *Posttest*

Urine

On the requisition slip and specimen container, write the time and date of the start and completion of the test.

Serum and Urine

Write the date of the last menstrual period on the requisition slip.

The specimen must be delivered to the laboratory without delay.

✓ QUALITY CONTROL
If there is a delay before analysis, the laboratory must refrigerate the urine and freeze the serum.

M

• SERUM, URINE

Synonym: Mg⁺

NORMAL VALUES

SERUM
Adult: 1.3–2.1 mEq/L *or* SI 0.65–1.05 µmol/L
Child
12–20 years: 1.56 ± 0.21 mEq/L *or* SI 0.78 ± 0.11 µmol/L
6–12 years: 1.56 ± 0.18 mEq/L *or* SI 0.78 ± 0.09 µmol/L
5 months–6 years: 1.65 ± 0.23 mEq/L *or* SI 0.83 ± 0.12 µmol/L
Infant newborn–4 days: 1.2–1.8 mEq/L *or* SI 0.6–0.9 µmol/L

URINE
7.3–12.2 mg/dl *or* SI 3–5 µmd day

Purpose of the Test

The measurement of serum magnesium helps to evaluate electrolyte disorders, hypocalcemia, hypokalemia, and acid-base imbalance. It is also used to monitor patients who have cardiac disorders because of low magnesium levels. The test is also performed to monitor the pregnant patient with severe toxemia during the intravenous administration of magnesium sulfate.

When the serum value is abnormal, the urine is usually tested to obtain additional data. One of the problems of urine testing is that there is little agreement regarding the normal range of urine values. Because the normal values vary among laboratories and geographic regions, the reference value of a particular laboratory may vary from the value listed in this text.

Procedure

Serum

A red-topped tube is used to obtain 1 ml of venous blood.

Urine

A 24-hour specimen is collected in a large plastic, acid-wash container.

✓ QUALITY CONTROL

The tourniquet should be applied for no longer than 1 minute to avoid venous stasis. Venipuncture technique must be smooth, with a blood flow that fills the vacuum tube readily. If there is stasis or if the blood has excessive turbulence because of flawed venipuncture technique, the hemolysis of erythrocytes will cause a false elevation of the results.

Findings

Increase in Serum

Advanced renal failure
Addison's disease
Administration of multiple magnesium sulfate enemas
Excessive ingestion of magnesium-containing antacids
Magnesium sulfate infusion therapy

Decrease in Serum

Early renal disease
Inadequate dietary intake
Chronic glomerulonephritis
Malabsorption
Chronic alcoholism
Prolonged nasogastric drainage
Hypercalcemia
Severe burns
Pancreatitis
Hypoparathyroidism
Hemodialysis therapy
Hyperaldosteronism
Pregnancy
Cisplatin therapy
Prolonged hyperalimentation
Prolonged intravenous therapy
Diabetic ketoacidosis (during treatment)

Increase in Urine

Chronic renal disease
Addison's disease
Chronic alcoholism
Bartter's syndrome
Ingestion of excess magnesium
Cisplatin therapy
Diuretic therapy

Decrease in Urine

Advanced kidney failure
Acute or chronic diarrhea
Diabetic acidosis
Starvation
Pancreatitis
Dehydration
Primary aldosteronism
Malabsorption

Interfering Factors

Serum	*Urine*
Venous stasis	Contact of urine with metal
Hemolysis	Loss of part of the urine specimen
	Failure to refrigerate the specimen

Nursing Implementation

• *Pretest*

Serum

Instruct the patient to fast from food and fluids for 8 hours before the test.

• *Posttest*

Serum

Send the specimen to the laboratory, without delay.

> ✓ QUALITY CONTROL
> To avoid the clumping of erythrocytes and invalid test results, the blood must be centrifuged quickly. The serum must then be refrigerated until it is analyzed.

• *Pretest*

Urine

Instruct the patient to use the special laboratory container to collect the urine. If a bedpan or urinal is used for voiding, it must be made of plastic, not metal.

To begin the test, instruct the patient to void and discard the 8 a.m. specimen. For the next 24 hours, all urine is saved, including the 8 a.m. specimen of the next morning.

Instruct the patient to refrigerate the specimen container throughout the test period.

• *Posttest*

Urine

Label the bottle with the patient's name and the time and date of the start and completion of the test.

Arrange for prompt transport of the chilled specimen to the laboratory.

MAGNETIC RESONANCE IMAGING	• MAGNETIC FIELD SCAN

Synonyms: MRI, nuclear magnetic resonance, NMR

N O R M A L   V A L U E S

No structural or anatomic abnormalities are noted.

Purpose of the Test

An MRI is a *noninvasive* imaging technique that uses a large, powerful magnet and radiofrequency coil to obtain cross-sectional images of body tissue. MRI is used to assess anatomic structures, organs, and soft tissue. It can visualize tumors, strictures, abscesses, atrophy, malformations, edema, and obstructions, including arterial narrowing. A cardiac MRI can noninvasively evaluate ejection fraction, cardiac output, and patency of proximal coronary arteries. It can assist in differentiating benign and malignant growths and may be used to stage cancers and evaluate response to treatment of malignancy.

Procedure

The patient enters the tube of the MRI machine, which contains a circular magnet and a radiofrequency coil. In the presence of the magnetic field and radio wave stimulation, there are changes in and movement of tissue protons. These movements are converted by computer to precise images of the tissue in any plane selected. The total time for test completion is about 90 minutes.

Findings

Tumor
Abscess
Stricture
Inflammation
Stenosis
Edema
Thrombus
Fluid collection
Embolus
Bleeding or hemorrhage
Arterio-venous malformation
Organ atrophy

Interfering Factors

Claustrophobia
Jewelry or metal in the magnetic field
Metallic implant in the body
Uncooperative behavior
Permanent pacemaker
Implanted cardioverters
Aneurysm clips

Nursing Implementation

- *Pretest*

Ask the patient if there is a history of any metallic implant having been placed in the body.

Assess for the presence of a permanent pacemaker. Cardiac pacemakers frequently contain ferromagnetic material and a magnetically activated relay switch. In addition, pacemaker leads may act as antennae, inducing electric shock.

Explain the procedure and sensations that the patient will experience. Obtain written consent from the patient or person legally designated to make the patient's health care decisions.

To help minimize anxiety, encourage the patient to have a friend or relative stay during the procedure.

To help minimize the emotional discomfort, encourage the patient to use relaxation strategies.

Instruct the patient how to obtain help while inside the machine.

Sedatives are usually used for the infant or child less than 3 years old, particularly when the scan requires an extended period of immobility. Administer the prescribed sedative. The medication is usually chloral hydrate or phenobarbital.

- *During the Test*

Instruct the patient to remain motionless on the narrow table during the test.

- *Posttest*

If sedatives were administered, monitor the vital signs on a regular basis until the patient is responsive and awake.

No other special nursing measures are needed.

✓ QUALITY CONTROL

Utilization of MRI in assessing cardiac function is limited because of the heart's constant motion. To control for the motion, various ''gating'' techniques are used to obtain an image at a certain time during the cardiac cycle. This technique is dependent on timing the R wave on the ECG or the patient's arterial wave form; therefore, is not reliable if the patient has an irregular rhythm.

✓ QUALITY CONTROL

The MRI produces a magnetic field, which can cause metal objects, such as pens, IV poles, and oxygen tanks, to become projectiles. Many MRI units have metal detectors to screen patients and personnel entering the area.

MAMMOGRAPHY (MAMMOGRAM)   •   RADIOGRAPHY

NORMAL VALUES

The breast tissue is within normal limits.

Purpose of the Test

This test screens for breast cancer and it investigates a symptomatic change in the breast tissue. It helps differentiate between benign and malignant diseases of the breast.

Procedure

X-ray films of each breast are taken from different angles.

Findings

Benign cyst
Microcalcifications
Fibroadenoma
Malignancy of the breast

Interfering Factors

Jewelry and clothing
Scar tissue from previous surgery
Body powders
Creams
Deodorants

Nursing Implementation

• *Pretest*

Instruct the patient not to use body creams, powders, and deodorants on the day of the test. The metallic elements in
these products interfere with visualization of the tissues.

Instruct the patient to remove all jewelry and clothing above
the waist. The examining gown is put on with the opening
to the front.

MANTOUX SKIN TEST (PPD) • SKIN TEST

NORMAL VALUES

Negative: Induration <5 mm

Purpose of the Test

The Mantoux test screens for tuberculosis exposure, a previously
healed tubercular infection, or active tuberculosis disease.

Procedure

An injection of 0.1 ml of purified protein derivitive (PPD) solution is injected intradermally, with an assessment of the skin site
48 to 72 hours later.

Findings

Positive

Tuberculosis infection

Interfering Factors

Immunosuppressive disorder
Steroid therapy
Previous tuberculosis infection
Previous vaccination with BCG vaccine

Nursing Implementation

• *Pretest*

This test is contraindicated when the patient has a previous
positive skin test, a history of tuberculosis, or immunization
with BCG vaccine.

Ensure that epinephrine hydrochloride, 1:1000, is at hand. There is a small risk of an anaphylactic reaction to the PPD solution.

• *During the Test*

Draw up 0.1 ml of the PPD solution in a tuberculin syringe.

On the inner aspect of the forearm, select a site that is free of skin eruption, infection, and excess hair. Cleanse the test site with alcohol.

Hold the skin taut and introduce the needle between the layers of skin. As the PPD solution is injected, a wheal or blister-like formation is created.

• *Posttest*

Record the Mantoux test administration in the patient's record. Include the site of the injection, the dose and strength of the solution, the time, and the date.

Instruct the patient that normal activities including bathing can be resumed. If the test site itches, it must not be scratched or rubbed. To read the result, the patient must return in 48 to 72 hours.

To read the test result, inspect and palpate the test site for a red, raised area of tissue reaction. Use a millimeter tape to measure the diameter of a raised area. Record the measurement.

A measurement of 5 to 9 mm of induration is considered a borderline result, and a repeat test with a stronger concentration of PPD is indicated. Induration of 10 mm or more is considered a positive result.

MIXED VENOUS BLOOD GASES • VENOUS

Synonyms: None

NORMAL VALUES

pH: 7.33–7.43 *or* SI 7.33–7.43
Pco_2: 41–51 mm Hg *or* SI 5.3–6.0 kPa
HCO_3^-: 24–28 mm Hg *or* SI 24–28 µmol/L
Pvo_2: 35–49 mm Hg
Svo_2: 60–80%

Purpose of the Test

Mixed venous blood gases are obtained to assess the O_2 supply and tissue O_2 consumption. Mixed venous blood gases provide a method for evaluating the dynamic balance between O_2 supply and O_2 delivery to the body. Since the organs of the body use various amounts of O_2, mixed venous blood gases measure the blood in the pulmonary artery, which contains the venous return from all the body systems. Arterial blood gases reflect what is available for body use (supply), whereas venous blood gases tell how well the body delivered and used this supply. Changes in Svo_2 indicate a need to determine which factor in O_2 supply and delivery is abnormal: cardiac output, hemoglobin level, tissue O_2 consumption, or Sao_2.

The Svo_2 is used to evaluate the response to nursing care. For an unstable patient, changes in position, bathing, suctioning, and so forth can increase O_2 consumption, resulting in a corresponding lowering of the Svo_2. If the Svo_2 falls to less than 60% or varies by 10% from the patient's baseline for longer than 3 minutes (10 minutes after suctioning), a full assessment of the patient is needed, including a cardiac output determination.

Procedure

A mixed venous sample may be obtained in a heparinized syringe from the distal port of the pulmonary artery catheter, or continuous Svo_2 may be assessed from a fiberoptic pulmonary artery catheter attached to an oximeter.

Findings

Increase in Svo_2	*Decrease in Svo_2*
Anesthesia	Anemia
Cyanide toxicity	Anxiety
High Fio_2	Bleeding
Hypothermia	Cardiogenic shock
Left-to-right shunt	Congestive heart failure
Neuromuscular blockade	Fever
Relaxation	Hyperthermia
Sepsis, sleep	Hypovolemia
Vasodilation	Inadequate Fio_2
	Large burns
	Pulmonary disease
	Multiple trauma

Decrease in Svo$_2$ (cont.)
Position changes
Seizures
Severe pain
Shivering
Suctioning

Interfering Factors

Inadequate perfusion
Poorly positioned pulmonary artery catheter

Nursing Implementation

Care is based on the technique used. With a random mixed venous blood gas determination, use the procedure that follows.

• *Pretest*

Explain the procedure to the patient.
Assess the hemodynamic monitoring system.
Gather equipment: one 3-ml syringe, two 10-ml syringes, a syringe cap, heparin, and ice.

• *During the Test*

Wear gloves.
Draw up 1 ml of heparin into the 3-ml syringe and draw back to coat the barrel. Expel heparin, leaving heparin in the needle.
Attach an empty 10-ml syringe to the sampling stopcock at the distal port of the pulmonary artery catheter.
Turn the stopcock off to the infusion solution.
Aspirate 5 ml into the syringe to clear the distal line of solution. Close the stopcock to the infusion and syringe.
Remove the syringe and discard. In special situations, such as in neonates, the blood is saved and returned to the patient after the sample is drawn.
Attach the 3-ml heparinized syringe to the stopcock.
Open the stopcock to the syringe and aspirate blood slowly.
Close the stopcock, remove the 3-ml syringe, and expel any air bubbles. Cap the syringe.
Gently roll the syringe in your hand to mix heparin and blood.

Place on ice.

Attach a 10-ml syringe to the stopcock. Open the stopcock to the solution and flush to clear the stopcock of blood.

Turn solution off to the stopcock port used to obtain the sample and cap the sampling port.

Flush the line and ensure the patency of the distal port. Check the monitor for pulmonary artery waveform.

Send blood to the laboratory immediately; clearly indicate on the slip that the blood is a mixed venous sample.

Obtain and send an ABG sample, if ordered.

• *Posttest*

Compare ABG and mixed venous blood gas samples.

With continuous Svo_2 monitoring, a special pulmonary artery catheter is inserted with Svo_2 sampling capability.

• *During the Test*

Attach Svo_2 port to the oximeter.

Calibrate the oximeter when the catheter is inserted and once a day while it is in the patient.

Calibration or recalibration is needed if there is a 4% or greater difference between the mixed venous sample sent to the laboratory and the Svo_2 reading on the oximeter.

Set alarm parameter at plus and minus 10% of the displayed Svo_2.

Adjust alarms as the patient's Svo_2 varies or the oximeter is recalibrated.

If intensity alarm signals, check catheter placement and patency. Check for air bubbles in the system or kinking of the catheter. Reposition the patient. Flush the catheter if needed.

Document hourly Svo_2 readings.

MYOGLOBULIN • Serum

N O R M A L   V A L U E S

40–180 mg/dl *or* SI <55 ng/ml

Purpose of the Test

Myoglobulin is an oxygen-binding protein found in skeletal, smooth, and cardiac muscle. Its levels may be used with cardiac enzymes to diagnosis myocardial infarction, evaluate muscle injury, or assess polymyositis.

Procedure

A venipuncture is performed to obtain 5 ml of blood in a red-topped tube.

Findings

Increase

Myocardial infarction
Muscle injury or breakdown
Polymyositis
Renal failure
Open-heart surgery
Exhaustive exercises

Interfering Factors

Trauma to skeletal muscle (limits usefulness in diagnosing myocardial infarction)
Recent administration of radioactive material if RIA method of analysis is used.

Nursing Implementation

Similar to other venipuncture.

NASOPHARYNGEAL AND THROAT CULTURE	• SECRETIONS

N O R M A L   V A L U E S

Negative: Normal flora in the nasopharynx or oropharynx

Purpose of the Test

The nasopharyngeal culture is performed to identify the bacteria that cause upper respiratory tract infection. The throat culture identifies the bacteria that cause infection of the oropharynx, pharynx, and tonsils. Both are used to screen for an asymptomatic carrier of infection.

Procedure

Nasopharyngeal Culture

A sterile, flexible wire swab is used to collect a specimen from the posterior nasopharynx. For a *fungeal culture*, scrapings of the cells are taken. In the culture for *Staphylococcus aureus,* a sterile, cotton-tipped applicator stick is used for the collection of a specimen from the anterior nasopharynx.

Throat Culture

A sterile, cotton-tipped swab is used to obtain a specimen of exudate from the throat.

In each case, the specimen is then placed in a sterile culture tube and capped tightly.

Findings

Positive

Nasopharynx	Throat
Pharyngitis	Pharyngitis
Thrush	Thrush

Nasopharynx (cont.)

Scarlet fever
Pertussis
Diphtheria
S. aureus carrier

Throat (cont.)

Scarlet fever
Pertussis
Diphtheria
Gonococcal infection

Interfering Factors

Antibiotic therapy
Improper technique in specimen collection
Contamination of the specimen

Nursing Implementation

- *Pretest*

If possible, obtain the specimen before antibiotics are started.
Inform the patient that the sterile wire or swab will be put into
the back of the nose or throat. Any mild discomfort disappears after the swab is removed.
In cases of acute epiglottitis or suspected diphtheria, do not
perform a nasopharyngeal culture until prepared to establish an alternate airway if needed. If diphtheria or gonorrhea is suspected, notify the laboratory in advance. Special
culture medium and transport are needed.

- *During the Test*

Help the patient sit up and tilt the head back. Use a light to
visualize the area to be cultured.

Nasopharynx

Insert the sterile wire through the nasal passage into the nasopharynx. Allow the wire to remain for about 5 seconds. The
patient may gag.
S. aureus culture: Insert the sterile wire 1 inch into the nares
and rotate it against the nasal mucosa.

Throat

Use a tongue blade to depress the tongue.
The sterile swab is used to rub the areas of exudate and inflammation in the oropharynx and on the tonsils.

✓ QUALITY CONTROL
Do not allow the swab or wire to touch the tongue, cheeks, uvula, or unintended parts of the nasopharynx. Poor technique causes contamination of the specimen.

• *Posttest*

On the requisition slip, write patient's name, age, time, date, and specific site used to obtain the culture specimen. Include the suspected clinical diagnosis and any current antibiotic therapy.

Arrange for prompt transport of the specimen to the laboratory.

✪ **COMPLICATION ALERT** ✪ In suspected cases of acute epiglottitis or diphtheria, assess the patient for a possible laryngospasm immediately after the throat culture has been obtained. Prepare to support oxygenation and assist with the establishment of an airway as needed.

NUCLEAR SCAN (ISOTOPE SCAN)	• RADIONUCLIDE STUDY

N O R M A L   V A L U E S

There is a normal uptake, distribution, and excretion of the radionuclide by the targeted organ or tissue. There is no abnormality of structure or function in the targeted organ.

Purpose of the Test

A nuclear scan is used to assess the physiologic function and assist in the localization and diagnosis of abnormality in a designated organ or tissue.

Procedure

A radiopharmaceutical designed to concentrate in the target organ is administered to the patient. A gamma camera or scintillation scanner records the radioactive emissions. These emissions are then converted by computer to images that correspond to the location, distribution, and concentration of the radionuclide in the targeted organ or tissue.

Findings

Organ atrophy or fibrosis
Cyst
Tumor
Metastatic lesion
Inflammation
Abscess
Acogenital defect
Obstruction of a duct
Hyperactivity of function
Hematoma
Traumatic disruption of tissue
Vascular obstruction
Ischemia or necrosis of tissue

Interfering Factors

Failure to follow specific pretest dietary or medication restrictions
Recent intake of iodine

Nursing Implementation

• *Pretest*

Obtain a written consent.

Provide the pretest patient instructions, which vary for each scan. Some scans have dietary restrictions to prevent an increase in the circulation to the liver or intestines. Many medications interfere with the absorption of the radiopharmaceutical. Often, after consultation with the patient's physician, medications are withheld and the patient remains under medical supervision during the period of the test.

If the scan involves the uptake of radioactive iodine (iodine-123, iodine-125, or iodine-131), instruct the patient to avoid the intake of iodine from food (shellfish, kelp preparations, and some vitamins) and medication sources (some cough medicines, Lugol's solution) for 3 to 5 days before the test.

On the day of the test, assist the patient in removing all clothing, jewelry, and metal objects. A hospital gown is worn.

Provide reassurance regarding the scanning process. Other than the venipuncture, the procedure is painless. If the patient is anxious, a family member or friend can be in the room during the scanning procedure.

- *During the Test*

Instruct the patient to remain in the preestablished position while a bolus dose of radionuclide is administered intravenously and during the scanning process, which may begin immediately after the injection.

- *Posttest*

As with the handling of all body fluids or waste products, wear gloves to dispose of any urine or feces and then wash your hands. The radionuclide is excreted in urine and feces for several days, although the radioactivity level is minimal after a few hours. The body wastes can be disposed of in the toilet.

Instruct the patient to wash his or her hands after voiding or a bowel movement. Reassure the patient that the amount of radioactivity is negligible, but it can remain on the hands unless they are washed.

O

OCCULT BLOOD, STOOL (FECAL OCCULT BLOOD TEST, FOBT)

• FECES

NORMAL VALUES

Negative for fecal occult blood

Purpose of the Test

This test detects fecal occult blood from a gastrointestinal source. It is used as a screening tool for an early diagnosis of bowel cancer. Positive results are followed up with additional diagnostic testing to locate the source and cause of bleeding.

Procedure

Two stool samples each day for 3 days (total = 6) are collected in plastic containers.

Findings

Colon cancer
Arteriovenous malformation in the colon
Benign polyps of the colon
Esophageal varices
Mallory-Weiss tear
Hiatal hernia
Gastritis
Peptic ulcer
Intussusception
Dysentery
Parasitic disease
Crohn's disease
Kaposi's sarcoma
Diverticular disease

Interfering Factors

Recent dietary intake of animal protein
Vegetables with peroxidase and high concentrations of
vitamin C
Failure to refrigerate the specimen

Nursing Implementation

• *Pretest*

Instruct the patient to avoid the following foods for 2 days before the test and during the test period: red meat, turnips,
and horseradish. Citrus juice can be taken in limited quantity only.
Inform the patient to discontinue aspirin, nonsteroidal anti-
inflammatory drugs, and alcohol until the test is completed.

> ✓ QUALITY CONTROL
> Animal protein and vegetables add to the peroxidase measured
> in the test. Ascorbic acid inhibits the peroxidase activity. These
> alterations falsely affect test results.

Instruct the patient regarding correct collection procedure.
There should be no water, urine, or paper mixed in with
the specimen. Each daily stool collection is placed in a separate plastic container with a lid. The specimens are refrigerated until taken to the laboratory.

OSMOLALITY • PLASMA OR SERUM, URINE

Synonyms: None

N O R M A L   V A L U E S

SERUM
Adult: 285–319 mOsm/kg H_2O *or* SI 280–395 µmol/kg
Children: 270–290 mOsm/kg H_2O *or* SI 270–290 µmol/kg

URINE
With normal diet and fluid intake: 500–800 mOsm/kg H_2O
or SI 500–800 µmol/kg H_2O
Range: 50–1400 mOsm/kg H_2O *or* SI 50–1400 µmol/kg H_2O

Purpose of the Test

Osmolality is a measure of the number of particles dissolved in a solution. In the blood, the osmolality is created by sodium, chloride, bicarbonate, proteins, glucose, and urea dissolved in the plasma. Osmolality will be affected by an increase or decrease in fluid volume or by an increase or decrease in blood particles.

Serum

Plasma osmolality is determined to assess the person's fluid status and identify ADH abnormalities.

Urine

Urine osmolality is determined to assess the ability of the kidneys to concentrate or dilute urine and to identify ADH abnormalities. Urine osmolality varies based on the person's fluid status and the metabolic waste products being excreted. If the patient is overhydrated, the urinary osmolality decreases as output increases. If the person is dehydrated, the urine osmolality increases as the output decreases. Urine osmolality is based on the concentration ability of the kidneys and the serum osmolality.

Procedure

Serum

Venipuncture is performed to obtain 1 ml of blood in a red-top tube. Osmolality is measured by the freezing point depression of solution using an osmometer or cryoscope or by the vapor pressure or dew point osmometer.

Urine

Ten ml of urine is collected in a sterile container and is sent to the laboratory.

Findings

Serum

Increase	Decrease
Alcoholism	Addison's disease
Aldosteronism	Fluid overload
Dehydration	Liver failure with ascites
Diabetes insipidus (DI)	Syndrome of inappropriate
Diabetic ketoacidosis	antidiuretic hor-
High-protein diets	mone(SIADH)

Hypercalcemia
Hyperglycemia
Hypernatremia
Hyperkalemia

Urine

Increase

Addison's disease
Azotemia
Cirrhosis of the liver
Dehydration
Diabetes mellitus
Diarrhea
Hyperglycemia
Hypernatremia
SIADH

Decrease

Aldosterone
DI
Glomerulonephritis
Hypocalcemia
Hyponatremia
Overhydration
Sickle cell anemia

Interfering Factors

Serum

Hemolysis of specimen
Medications (diuretics, mineralocorticoids)

Urine

Noncompliance with the nothing-by-mouth order
Glucosuria
Recent scans requiring radiopaque dyes
Medications (antibiotics, diuretics, volume expanders)

Nursing Implementation

Serum

The nursing actions are similar to those of other venipuncture procedures.

• *Pretest*

Urine

Instruct the patient not to eat or drink overnight before the urine is collected.

- *During the Test*

Urine

Obtain 10 ml of urine in a sterile container.

- *Posttest*

Urine

Send to the laboratory immediately.

OVA AND PARASITES (STOOL FOR O & P) • FECES

NORMAL VALUES

Negative

Purpose of the Test

The microscopic examination of the feces is used to identify the presence of specific parasites in the intestinal tract.

Procedure

Stool Collection

Collect a small sample of feces directly into a clean, wide-mouthed container and close the lid. A common requirement is to collect one specimen each day for 3 days.

Perianal Swab

Transparent tape is placed on a tongue depressor, sticky side out. Press the tape firmly on the perianal skin. Place the tape on a glass slide, sticky side down.

Findings

Amebiasis
Giardiasis
Cryptosporidiosis
Tapeworm
Ascariasis
Hookworm
Pinworm

Interfering Factors

Antibiotic therapy
Contamination of the specimen
Barium sulfate
Mineral oil
Castor oil
Antacids
Antidiarrheal medication

Nursing Implementation

- *Pretest*

Schedule this test prior to any barium studies.
Instruct the patient regarding correct collection procedure.
   The feces should not be removed from the toilet bowl.

- *Posttest*

Place the lid on the specimen container. Remove gloves and
   wash your hands thoroughly.

✓ QUALITY CONTROL
Intestinal parasites are easily transmitted by the fecal-oral route
or by contact with the skin. Precautions are taken to prevent infection from poor hygiene practices.

Include the time and date of the collection on the laboratory
   slip and the container. Send the specimen to the laboratory
   immediately because the examination of the specimen must
   begin within 30 to 60 minutes.

✓ QUALITY CONTROL
Time delay and exposure to heat or cold temperatures will kill
any trophozoites or cysts.

P

N O R M A L   V A L U E S

Bethesda system classification: Normal; within normal limits

Purpose of the Test

This test detects inflammation, premalignant changes, and malignancy or infection of the vagina and cervix. It is also used to evaluate the response of the cervix to chemotherapy or radiotherapy in the treatment of cancer.

Procedure

Using a vaginal speculum to enhance visibility, secretions and cells from the cervix and vagina are collected. The fluid and tissue scrapings are placed on glass slides and sprayed with or immersed in a fixative.

> ✓ QUALITY CONTROL
> The speculum is not lubricated before insertion because the lubricant would interfere with the microscopic viewing of the slides. The fixative must be applied promptly to prevent drying of the cells.

Findings

Cervical dysplasia
Cervical intraepithelial neoplasia
Infection
Endometriosis
Condyloma
Human papillomavirus
Lymphogranuloma venereum
Carcinoma in situ
Adenocarcinoma

Interfering Factors

Menstruation
Recent douching
Vaginal infection or medication
Recent sexual intercourse
Drying of the specimen
Inadequate specimen

Nursing Implementation

• *Pretest*

Schedule the test when the patient is not menstruating.
Instruct the patient to refrain from sexual intercourse, douching, and vaginal medication for 48 hours before the test.
Prior to the examination, instruct the patient to void.

• *During the Test*

Place patient in lithotomy position with the legs supported by stirrups.
After the fixative is dry, identify each slide with the patient's name.

• *Posttest*

On the requisition slip, write the patient's name, age, date of last menstrual period, and the source of the specimen. Include the pertinent clinical history.
If the result is abnormal, the patient often requires additional information about the meaning of the results and the follow-up measures. She may experience anxiety, confusion, or emotional upset.

PARATHYROID HORMONE • SERUM

Synonyms: Parathormone, PTH

NORMAL VALUES

(Interpreted in relation to serum calcium levels)
Intact parathyroid hormone: 10–50 pg/ml *or* SI 1.1–5.3 pmol/L
N-terminal fraction: 8–24 pg/ml *or* SI 0.8–2.5 pmol/L
C-terminal fraction: 0–340 pg/ml *or* SI 0–35.8 pmol/L

Purpose of the Test

A parathyroid hormone determination is performed to diagnose suspected parathyroid disorders. It may be performed to differentiate between clinical diagnoses that result in calcium and phosphate abnormalities.

Procedure

Parathyroid hormone is frequently measured by RIA, which can measure biologically active intact parathyroid hormone. This fraction represents only a small portion of the total parathyroid hormone. Alternatively, RIA can measure C-terminal or N-terminal portions of the hormone. Two venous samples, 3 ml each in red-topped tubes, are needed.

Findings

Increase	*Decrease*
Hyperparathyroidism	Hypoparathyroidism
	Lung, kidney, pancreatic, or ovarian cancer

Interfering Factors

Noncompliance with fasting requirements
Elevated lipid levels

Nursing Implementation

The actions of the nurse are similar to those carried out in other venipuncture procedures.

• *Pretest*

Instruct the patient not to eat or drink for 12 hours before the test.

• *Posttest*

The patient may resume a normal diet.

PATCH TEST, SKIN • SKIN SENSITIVITY TESTS

Synonyms: None

N O R M A L   V A L U E S

Negative: No abnormal skin reactions are noted.

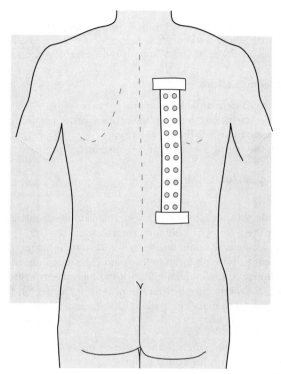

Figure 4. Patch Test. Various allergens are applied to the skin of the patient's back. Those allergens that cause an allergic skin response are identified as the sources of contact dermatitis.

Purpose of the Test

This test is used to determine the cause of contact dermatitis by identifying the particular allergen. It is also used to differentiate contact dermatitis from other causes of eczematous disease.

Procedure

Samples of selected allergens used by the patient or a number of standard allergens are taped to the patient's skin for 48 hours (Fig. 4). The readings of the results are performed at 48 hours and again at 72 hours to 7 days, as prescribed.

Findings

A positive reaction is a red, raised, pruritic area of skin where a particular allergen was placed. An undecided result is a red flat lesion. A negative reaction demonstrates no change.

Interfering Factors

Concurrent dermatitis from another source
Exposure of the patch site to water or excessive perspiration
Inaccurate interpretation of the results
Inaccurate timing for the reading of results

Nursing Implementation

- *Pretest*

Schedule this test after the acute dermatitis has subsided and after the treatment with corticosteroids has ceased.

If the products the patient uses are to be tested, instruct the patient to bring them in beforehand. The patch test must be prepared and a detailed list of the ingredients written.

Obtain a signed consent from the patient or the person legally designated to make the patient's health care decisions.

- *During the Test*

Tape the allergen patch to the patient's upper back between the scapula and the spinal column.

Make a diagram on paper to identify the location of each allergen.

- *Posttest*

Instruct the patient to refrain from showers and physical exercise during the next 48 hours. Water and perspiration would loosen the tape of the patch.

Inform the patient that the itching is usually caused by the tape. If, however, there is burning or pain under one of the discs of allergen, it may be removed from that one area.

Instruct the patient to return in 48 hours for the first evaluation of the results. The patch is removed at that time. After a 30-minute to 1-hour wait, the skin is assessed for any reaction in the area of the patch. Instruct the patient to return for the second appointment to reevaluate the skin. This is scheduled to be performed 72 hours to 7 days after the patch is applied.

Inform the patient that exercise and showers are permitted while waiting for the second evaluation, but there can be no use of soap and no scrubbing, scratching, or rubbing the skin in the test area.

PERICARDIOCENTESIS • PATHOLOGY

Synonym: Pericardial fluid analysis

NORMAL VALUES

Fluid is sterile, clear, or straw-colored.

Purpose of the Test

Pericardiocentesis is a diagnostic and therapeutic procedure in which the pericardial space is accessed with a needle or cannula, and fluid is aspirated. For diagnostic purposes, the fluid is then analyzed. For therapeutic purposes, either fluid is drained on a one-time basis or a catheter is left in place for 1 to 48 hours (rarely, it may be kept in for 72 hours).

Analysis of pericardial fluid is performed to determine the cause of and appropriate therapy for acute pericarditis, subacute effusive-constrictive pericarditis, neoplastic pericardial disease, and pericardial effusion of unknown cause.

Procedure

A pericardiocentesis for diagnostic purposes is not an emergency situation and can be performed in the controlled environment of an operating room or special procedure room. The procedure begins after a skin preparation and infiltration of a local anesthetic, usually 1% lidocaine without epinephrine. A small incision is made in the skin, the site being determined by the desired approach. A needle is inserted through the incision until a "popping" or "giving" sensation is felt as the pericardium is entered. Traditionally, an electrocardiographic lead is attached to the pericardiocentesis needle. As the needle advances, a chest lead on the ECG is recorded. When the heart is punctured, a zone of injury pattern is noted, and the needle is withdrawn slightly. Some physicians do not recommend this technique because poor electrocardiographic tracings prevent the zone of injury from being seen, which may lead to cardiac lacerations. The sign of injury on the ECG also may not occur if the needle infiltrates an area of fibrosis, a tumor, or infiltrative cardiomyopathy tissue. There is a possibility of ventricular fibrillation if the electrocardiograph is not grounded properly, there is electric leakage, or the individual performing the procedure accidentally touches the needle and electrocardiograph.

Once the needle is in position, approximately 20 ml of fluid is removed for analysis. If cytologic studies are performed, a heparinized container is necessary. The fluid is usually analyzed for color; hemoglobin concentration; hematocrit value; red blood cell, white blood cell, and differential counts; and protein and glucose determinations. In addition, gram stains and culture, fungal stains and culture, and cytologic studies are performed. Additional fluid is removed if viral and parasite studies, immunologic and serologic screens, or lipoelectrophoresis is planned.

If therapeutic pericardiocentesis is desired after the specimens are obtained, a catheter is inserted and positioned to allow drainage.

Findings

Bacterial, viral, or fungal infection
Malignancies

Interfering Factors

Pericardiocentesis requires a patient who is cooperative and who will lie still during the procedure. Uncooperative patients may require sedation. Those on anticoagulant therapy, with bleeding disorders or thrombocytopenia, are not appropriate candidates. If cultures of the fluid are planned, administration of antibiotics will affect the results.

Nursing Implementation

• Pretest

Ensure that an informed consent form has been signed.
Explain the procedure to the patient.
Check laboratory work for bleeding problems.
Obtain a baseline ECG if ordered.
Document baseline vital signs and heart sounds.
Take medication history to check for anticoagulant use.

The patient maintains a nothing-by-mouth status for 4 to 6 hours before the test.

Administer sedation as prescribed.

Shave site if necessary.

• *During the Test*

Position the patient. Usually a recumbent position is used, with the torso and head elevated 30 to 45 degrees.

Ensure that an intravenous infusion is present and patent.

Maintain patient on telemetry or cardiac monitor.

Frequent vital signs are taken.

Have a defibrillator and emergency drugs on hand.

Continue to reassure and support the patient, who will feel the local anesthetic being infiltrated and may experience a sharp pain when the pericardium is infiltrated.

• *Posttest*

The patient may return to pretest activities gradually if vital signs are stable.

Assess for recurrence of symptoms.

Observe for complications: laceration of coronary artery, cardiac chamber, ventricular fibrillation, pneumothorax and peritoneal puncture.

PERITONEAL FLUID ANALYSIS (PARACENTESIS)	• **PERITONEAL FLUID**

N O R M A L   V A L U E S

Appearance: clear, odorless, pale yellow, scanty
Ammonia: <50 µg/dl
Amylase: 138–404 amylase units/L
Bacteria/fungi: none
Cells: no malignant cells present
Glucose: 70–90 mg/dl *or* SI 3.89–4.99 µmol/L
Protein: 0.3–4.1 g/dl *or* SI 3–41 g/L
Red blood cells: none
White blood cells: <300 per µl *or* SI <300 x 10^6/L

Purpose of the Test

Peritoneal fluid analysis is used as part of the investigation for the cause of ascites. Laboratory examination may include cytologic study, chemistry analysis, and microbiologic examination.

Procedure

Under local anesthesia, a special needle or trocar is inserted into the abdominal cavity and fluid is removed. For cytologic examination, 50 to 250 ml of fluid is needed.

Findings

Peritonitis
Intestinal perforation
Rupture of the bowel, gallbladder, spleen, liver, or bladder
Cirrhosis
Pancreatitis
Hypoproteinemia
Benign or malignant tumor

Interfering Factors

Contamination of the fluid by urine, feces, blood, or bile
Pregnancy
Coagulation disorder
Intestinal obstruction
Adhesions
Uncooperative behavior
Portal hypertension

Nursing Implementation

• *Pretest*

Within 48 hours of the test, obtain the hematocrit, prothrombin time, partial thromboplastin time, and platelet values. Post the results in the chart.

Obtain a written consent.

Record baseline vital signs, temperature, weight, and measure of the abdominal girth.

Just prior to the procedure, have the patient void.

Position the patient in a full Fowler's position.

- *During the Test*

Reassure the patient, to alleviate fear. Some pain or a jolting sensation is felt when the needle or trocar penetrates the peritoneum. Encourage the patient to remain immobile during the procedure.

Assist with the collection of the fluid specimens.

Monitor vital signs every 15 minutes. Assess for shock.

Once the needle or trocar is removed, apply a small dressing.

- *Posttest*

Vital signs and abdominal girth measurement are recorded. Thereafter, the vital signs are taken every hour for 6 hours or until the patient is stable. The dressing is checked for excessive drainage or blood.

The nurse's note about the procedure describes the patient's tolerance of the test, the amount of fluid removed, and the color, odor, and characteristics of the fluid.

All specimens are appropriately labeled, including identification as a paracentesis specimen. The requisition slip states the specific laboratory analyses to be performed. All specimens are sent to the laboratory without delay.

✪ **COMPLICATION ALERT** ✪ The nurse assesses for signs of bleeding or hemorrhage (distended abdomen and ecchymosis at the needle site, flank, or back). If the bowel was perforated, there will be fever and a painful, acute abdomen. In cases of hemorrhage or bowel perforation, the patient may develop shock (hypotension, tachycardia, and diaphoresis).

PHENYLALANINE • BLOOD

Synonyms: Phe, PKU test, phenylalanine screening test, Guthrie screening test

N O R M A L   V A L U E S

GUTHRIE TEST
<2 mg/day/L *or* SI 121 µmol/L

FLUOROMETRY METHOD
Normal newborn: 1.2–3.4 mg/dl *or* SI 73–206 µmol/L
Premature newborn: 2–7.5 mg/dl *or* SI 121–454 µmol/L
Adult: 0.8–1.8 mg/dl *or* SI 48–109 µmol/L

Purpose of the Test

The blood phenylalanine test is performed to detect PKU and other causes of hyperphenylalaninemia. It is also used to monitor patients who have PKU and are being maintained on a phenylalanine-restricted diet.

Phenylketonuria (PKU) is an inherited disorder of amino acid metabolism that is characterized by elevated levels of phenylalanine and phenylpyruvic acid. Unless there is early detection and proper dietary intervention, the elevated blood level of phenylalanine will cause central nervous system damage and mental retardation. State laws require PKU testing of all newborns within a specified period. If the blood phenylalanine test is performed in the first 24 hours of life, the test should be repeated after feeding has begun. The repeat test would greatly reduce the chance of a false-negative result.

✓ QUALITY CONTROL

Premature or low-birth-weight infants have higher serum values than do full-term infants of normal weight. This false-positive serum elevation is caused by immaturity of the liver. Antibiotics also interfere with the Guthrie's method of analysis and cause a false-positive result.

Procedure

A heelstick puncture is used to obtain a few drops of blood. The blood sample is collected by capillary tube, PKU card, or filter paper. The circles are filled by blotting the blood onto the paper.

✓ QUALITY CONTROL

With the filter paper or card, only one side of the paper is blotted to fill the circles. The paper should not be turned over to soak the other side. Cord blood cannot be used for this test.

Findings

Increase

PKU
Severe burns
Hyperphenylalaninemia
Liver disease
Sepsis
Galactosemia

Interfering Factors

Little to no ingestion of milk
Insufficient quantity of blood
Antibiotics

Nursing Implementation

- *Pretest*

Ensure that the laboratory requisition slip includes the name,
date, time of the test, date of birth, and time of the first
milk feeding. The ideal time to screen the blood for phenylalanine is 48 to 72 hours after birth or 2 days after the newborn begins to feed.

Note the administration of antibiotics or blood transfusion.

- *Posttest*

Arrange for prompt transport of the specimen to the laboratory.

PHENYLALANINE	• URINE

Synonym: PKU urine test

N O R M A L   V A L U E S

FERRIC CHLORIDE METHOD
Green color is positive for phenylpyruvic acid.

PHENASTIX METHOD (URINE REAGENT DIP STRIP)
Persistent blue-gray to green-gray color is positive for phenylpyruvic acid.

Purpose of the Test

The urine phenylalanine test is used to assist in the detection of
hyperphenylalanemia, including PKU. The test is also used to
monitor the effect of dietary treatment for patients who have a
defect in amino acid metabolism.

PKU is one type of aminoaciduria. It is an inherited disorder of
amino acid metabolism caused by the absence of phenylalanine
hydroxylase. If the condition remains undetected or uncontrolled by dietary therapy, damage to the central nervous system
and mental retardation will occur. Phenylpyruvic acid is not pres-

ent in the urine at birth because there must first be an intake of protein from breast milk or infant formula. If the amino acid metabolism is impaired, there will be a rapid rise of phenylalanine in the blood. This can be detected readily by the serum phenylalanine test, which is the primary screening test for PKU. Once the serum level of phenylpyruvic acid rises to 10 to 20 mg/dl, the metabolite appears in the urine, but this takes 2 to 6 weeks to occur after birth.

Procedure

A freshly voided specimen of urine is collected in a plastic urine collection container.

Findings

PKU
Non-PKU hyperphenylalanemia

Interfering Factors

Inadequate labeling
Improper collection procedure
Diluted urine

Nursing Implementation

- *Pretest*

For testing infants and small children, teach the mother to apply the urine collection bag and transfer the urine to a collection container.

- *Posttest*

Ensure that the time and date of voiding are written on the label and requisition slip.

Arrange for the transport of the urine to the laboratory within 1 hour.

PHOSPHORUS • SERUM

Synonyms: P, inorganic phosphate, $PO_4^=$

NORMAL VALUES

Adult
  (12–60 years): 2.7–4.5 mg/dl *or* SI 0.87–1.45 μmol/L
  (>60 years): 2.3–3.7 mg/dl *or* SI 0.74–1.2 μmol/L

Child
  (2–12 years): 4.5–5.5 mg/dl or SI 1.45–1.78 µmol/L
  (10 days–2 years): 4.5–6.7 mg/dl or SI 1.45–2.16 µmol/L
Infant (0–10 days): 4.5–9 mg/dl or SI 1.45–2.91 µmol/L
Premature infant (1 week): 5.4–10.9 mg/dl or SI 1.74–3.52 µmol/L
Cord blood: 3.7–8.1 mg/dl or SI 0.85–1.5 µmol/L
  Plasma phosphate ($PO_4^=$)
Adult: 8.2–14.5 mg/dl or SI 0.85–1.5 µmol/L

Purpose of the Test

Serum phosphorus helps diagnose kidney disorders and acid-base imbalance. It is also used to detect disorders of calcium, bone, or endocrine origin. There is an inverse relationship between the serum levels of phosphorus and calcium. If the serum level of either mineral falls, the serum level of the other mineral rises.

Procedure

A red-topped tube is used to collect 1 ml of venous blood. For infants and small children, a heelstick puncture and capillary tube are used to collect a blood sample.

✓ QUALITY CONTROL
Venipuncture technique must be smooth, with a blood flow that fills the vacuum tube readily. If the blood has excessive turbulence because of flawed technique, the hemolysis of the erythrocytes will alter the results.

Findings

Increase

Renal failure
Cirrhosis of the liver
Hypovolemia
Pulmonary embolism
Dehydration
Diabetic ketoacidosis
Milk alkali syndrome
Vitamin D toxicity
Acromegaly
Respiratory acidosis

Decrease

Osteomalacia
Acute respiratory infection
Osteoblastic bone cancer
Prolonged intravenous glucose therapy
Acute gout
Prolonged nasogastric drainage
Vitamin D deficiency
Hyperparathyroidism

Increase (cont.)

Osteolytic metastatic bone
  cancer
Lactic acidosis
Sarcoidosis
Postanesthesia hyperthermia
Hypoparathyroidism

Decrease (cont.)

Renal tubular disease
Serum calcium elevation
Severe malabsorption
Vomiting
Diarrhea
Starvation
Sepsis
Respiratory alkalosis

Interfering Factors

Hemolysis
Carbohydrate-rich meals
Recent phosphate enema

Nursing Implementation

• *Pretest*

Schedule the test for early morning.
Instruct the patient to discontinue all food and fluids for
  8 hours before the test.

✓ QUALITY CONTROL
It is best to obtain a fasting specimen because carbohydrate intake and recent food intake tend to decrease the serum phosphate level. Early morning hours are used to obtain the blood
to avoid the diurnal fluctuations.

Do not administer a phosphate enema just prior to the test because some of the phosphate is absorbed by the colonic mucosa.

• *Posttest*

Arrange for prompt transport of the specimen.

✓ QUALITY CONTROL
A delay in centrifuge of the specimen results in a false rise of
the serum value.

PLETHYSMOGRAPHY, ARTERIAL • MANOMETRY

Synonyms: Pulse cuff recording, PCR, pneumoplethysmography

N O R M A L   V A L U E S

No evidence of arterial peripheral vascular disease; normal arterial waveform pattern

Purpose of the Test

Plethysmography is a noninvasive test that evaluates the arterial blood flow in the extremities. It detects the presence of peripheral arterial vascular disease.

Procedure

Plethysmograph cuffs and electrodes are applied to the extremity(ies). The cuffs are inflated at different levels on the extremities, and arterial waveforms are recorded. The total test takes about 30 minutes to complete.

Findings

Peripheral vascular disease
Arterial occlusive disease
Arterial embolus
Arterial trauma

Interfering Factors

Smoking
Caffeine
Alcohol
Cold room temperatures
Anxiety

Nursing Implementation

- *Pretest*

Explain the procedure to the patient and obtain written consent from the patient or person responsible for the patient's health care decisions.

Instruct the patient to refrain from smoking and alcohol and caffeine ingestion before the test because stimulants, depressants, and vasoconstrictive substances will alter the results.

Assist the patient in removing all clothing and putting on a hospital gown. Restrictive clothing can alter the circulatory flow to the extremities.

Place the patient in a supine position, with a pillow under the head.

Maintain a comfortable room temperature and dim the room lighting. Cool temperatures, anxiety, and muscle tension will alter the results.

Instruct the patient to refrain from talking and movement during the test.

• *During the Test*

The pressure cuffs are applied to both legs at the level of the upper thighs, above and below the knees, and above the ankles.

At the first cuff site, inflate the cuff to 75 mm Hg for 2 to 3 seconds and then lower the pressure to 65 mm Hg. Record four to five waveforms. Label the recording with the correct identification of the cuff level and right or left side. Repeat this procedure at each cuff site.

• *Posttest*

Deflate and remove the cuffs.
Wipe conductive gel off.

PLETHYSMOGRAPHY, VENOUS • MANOMETRY

Synonyms: Impedance plethysmography, venous cuff examination, maximal venous outflow test, occlusive phlebography

N O R M A L   V A L U E S

Normal waveform patterns with adequate venous capacity and maximum venous outflow; no evidence of deep vein thrombosis

Purpose of the Test

Venous plethysmography is used to detect deep vein thrombosis and to screen patients who are at high risk for the development of venous thrombosis. When a deep vein is obstructed by a thrombus, there is backup of the venous blood and engorgement of the distal vessel. Once the vein is compressed temporarily by the blood pressure cuff, there is further interruption of the blood flow. Increased engorgement of the distal vein cannot occur because the vein has already filled to capacity. On deflation of the cuff and release of the compression, there is resumption of only minimal venous blood flow because the thrombus continues to obstruct the lumen.

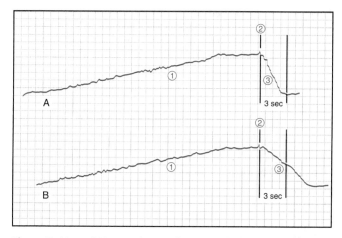

Figure 5. Normal Versus Abnormal Venous Plethysmographic Waveforms. *A,* The normal waveform (1) demonstrates complete venous capacitance, (2) release of the thigh cuff, and (3) rapid venous outflow that completes in 3 seconds. *B,* The abnormal waveform demonstrates (1) venous capacitance, (2) the release of the thigh cuff, and (3) slow venous outflow.

As the compression is applied to a normal vein, the venous plethysmography waveform pattern shows a gradual rise in height from the baseline. This phase is called venous capacitance and represents the filling of the distal vein to its fullest capacity. On release of the compression, the waveform drops rapidly and returns to baseline (Fig. 5). In an obstructed vein, the release of the pressure cuff relieves the venous compression, but there is limited venous outflow and slow emptying of the engorged vein. Correspondingly, the waveform demonstrates a limited, slow return to baseline.

Procedure

Plethysmograph cuffs and electrodes are applied to the thigh and calf to control and monitor venous blood flow. The cuffs are inflated, and the recorded waveforms demonstrate the filling of the vein to maximal capacity. On rapid release of the cuffs, the waveform demonstrates the venous outflow of the distal vein. The total time required to complete the test is 30 to 45 minutes.

Findings

Venous thrombosis
Thrombophlebitis
Venous obstruction (partial or complete)

Interfering Factors

Nicotine
Alcohol
Caffeine
Anxiety
Muscle tension
Uncooperative behavior
Compression of pelvic veins (tumor, tight bandages)
Low cardiac output
Shock
Arterial occlusive disease

Nursing Implementation

• *Pretest*

Inform the patient about the procedure and obtain written consent from the patient or person legally designated to make the patient's health care decisions.

Instruct the patient to refrain from smoking or ingesting alcohol or caffeine before the test because stimulants and relaxants will alter the test results.

Help the patient to remove all clothing and to put on a hospital gown. Any compression from restrictive clothing alters the venous circulation from the extremities. Maintain a comfortable room temperature and dim the lights because anxiety or muscle tension alters the results.

Place the patient in the supine position, with the legs elevated above the heart and supported by pillows. The affected leg and hip are externally rotated, and the knee is flexed.

Instruct the patient to refrain from movement or talking during the test.

• *During the Test*

Place blood pressure cuffs on the thigh and calf of the affected leg.

Apply the conductive gel and electrodes to the skin.

Inflate the cuff on the calf to 15 mm Hg of pressure. This cuff and electrode monitor the inflow of the venous system.

Inflate the cuff on the thigh to 55 mm Hg of pressure. This pressure level obstructs the venous outflow but allows the arterial flow to fill and engorge the distal vein segment.

Start the recorder to trace the waveform. Once the tracing has risen to its maximum and forms a plateau, the venous filling is completed.

Quickly release the pressure on the thigh cuff to open the venous outflow of the vein. The waveform pattern will continue and provide the linear recording of the return to the baseline reading.

Repeat the procedure until three to five waveforms are recorded.

Label the paper, correctly identifying the extremity.

Repeat the entire procedure on the opposite extremity to provide comparison data.

• *Posttest*

Remove the deflated cuffs and electrodes.

Wipe the conductive gel off the skin.

POTASSIUM • SERUM

Synonym: K$^+$

NORMAL VALUES

Adult: 3.5–5.1 mEq/L *or* SI 3.5–5.1 μmol/L
Child: 3.4–4.7 mEq/L *or* SI 3.4–4.7 μmol/L
Infant: 4.1–5.3 mEq/L *or* SI 4.1–5.3 μmol/L
Newborn: 3.7–5.9 mEq/L *or* SI 3.7–5.9 μmol/L
Premature (48 hours): 3.0–6.0 mEq/L *or* SI 3.0–6.0 μmol/L

Purpose of the Test

Serum potassium is used to evaluate electrolyte balance, acid-base balance, hypertension, renal disease or renal failure, and endocrine disease. It is used to monitor the patient receiving treatment for ketoacidosis as well as those receiving hyperalimentation, dialysis, diuretic therapy, and intravenous therapy. It is part of the routine blood chemistry screen or SMA (sequential multiple analyzer).

Procedure

A red- or green-topped tube is used to collect 5 to 7 ml of venous blood.

> ✓ QUALITY CONTROL
> Venipuncture technique must be smooth, with a blood flow that fills the tube readily. If the blood has excessive turbulence because of flawed technique, hemolysis of erythrocytes causes a false rise in the serum value.

Findings

Increase	*Decrease*
Rapid or excessive intravenous potassium replacement	Diuretic therapy
	Excessive sweating
Massive hemolysis	Intravenous fluid therapy without potassium replacement
Acidosis	
Dehydration	
Diabetic ketoacidosis	Fistula drainage
Acute renal failure	Bartter's syndrome
Traumatic crushing injury	Vomiting or diarrhea
Chronic renal failure	Alkalosis
Severe burns	Severe burns
Potassium-sparing diuretics	Aldosteronism
Addison disease	Renal tubular acidosis

Interfering Factors

Hemolysis

Nursing Implementation

• *Pretest*

In drawing the blood, it is preferable to avoid the use of a tourniquet. If the tourniquet is applied loosely, the fist should not be clenched. These measures prevent hemolysis of erythrocytes and a false elevation of the potassium value.

- Posttest

Arrange for transport of the specimen to the laboratory as quickly as possible.

> ✓ QUALITY CONTROL
> A clotted specimen causes a false elevation of the serum value when intracellular potassium is released into the extracellular serum.

PROGESTERONE (P₄) • SERUM

NORMAL VALUES

ADULT
Male: 13–97 ng/dl *or* SI 0.4–3.1 nmol/L
Female:
Follicular phase: 15–70 ng/dl *or* SI 0.5–2.2 nmol/L
Luteal phase: 200–2500 ng/dl *or* SI 6.4–79.5 nmol/L
Pregnant
7–13 weeks gestation: 1025–4400 ng/dl *or* SI 32.6–139.9 nmol/L
30–42 weeks gestation: 6500–22,900 ng/dl *or* SI 206.7–728.2 nmol/L

Purpose of the Test

Serum progesterone levels are used to determine ovulation and to assess the function of the corpus luteum, particularly in cases of habitual abortion or infertility.

Procedure

A red-topped tube is used to obtain 7 ml of venous blood.

Findings

Increase	*Decrease*
Congenital adrenal hyper-plasia	Threatened abortion
Molar pregnancy	Short luteal phase syndrome
Ovarian tumor	

Interfering Factors

Recent radioactive isotope scan

Nursing Implementation

• *Pretest*

Schedule this test before or at least 7 days after a nuclear scan.

> ✓ QUALITY CONTROL
> The radioisotopes of the scan would interfere with the radioim-munoassay method of analysis and the test results.

When a series of blood tests throughout the menstrual cycle is required, make sure that the patient understands the testing plan and schedule of test dates.

• *Posttest*

On the requisition slip, write the pertinent data, including the patient's sex, date of the patient's last menstrual period, and the trimester of pregnancy.

PROLACTIN (PRL, LACTOGENIC HORMONE)	• SERUM

N O R M A L   V A L U E S

Adult: 0–20 ng/ml *or* SI 0–20 µg/L
Pregnancy
  Third trimester: 34–306 ng/ml *or* SI 34–306 µg/L
  Lactating mother: <40 ng/ml *or* SI <40 µg/L

Purpose of the Test

The measurement of serum prolactin is used to evaluate oligor-rhea, amenorrhea, or galactorrhea. It may assist in the diagnosis of pituitary gland or hypothalamic dysfunction.

Procedure

A chilled, red-topped tube is used to collect 7 ml of venous blood 3 to 4 hours after arising from sleep.

✓ QUALITY CONTROL
To prevent hemolysis, venipuncture technique must be smooth, with a blood flow that fills the vacuum tube readily.

Findings

Increase

Hypothalamus-pituitary disease (sarcoidosis, metastatic cancer)
Prolactin-secreting pituitary tumor
Acromegaly
Hypothyroidism
Anorexia nervosa
Adrenal insufficiency

Decrease

Pituitary infarction or necrosis

Interfering Factors

Alcohol intake
Failure to fast in the pretest period
Recent radioactive isotope scan
Warming of the specimen
Hemolysis
Sleep disturbance

Nursing Implementation

- Pretest

Schedule this test before or at least 7 days after a nuclear scan.
Instruct the patient to abstain from alcohol for 24 hours and to fast from food for 8 hours before the blood is drawn.
Schedule the blood to be drawn between 8 a.m. and 10 a.m. or 3 to 4 hours after arising from sleep.

- Posttest

Ensure that the vial of blood is placed on ice. To maintain the cool temperature, arrange for prompt transport of the specimen to the laboratory.

PROSTATE BIOPSY • TISSUE BIOPSY

Synonyms: Core biopsy of the prostate gland, fine needle aspiration biopsy of the prostate gland

N O R M A L   V A L U E S

Normal prostate tissue with no evidence of tumor or infection

Purpose of the Test

A prostate biopsy is used to determine the cause of an enlarged prostate gland and to diagnose prostate cancer.

A biopsy of the prostate gland is indicated when there is a palpable nodule; alteration in size, shape, or texture of prostate tissue; abnormal findings on ultrasound of the prostate, or elevated blood levels of the tumor markers prostatic acid phosphatase or prostate-specific antigen.

Procedure

Using aseptic technique and local anesthesia to the perineum, a needle is inserted into the prostate tumor. Suction or a syringe is used to aspirate several samples of the tissue.

Findings

Cancer of the prostate gland
Benign prostatic hypertrophy
Lymphoma
Prostatitis

Interfering Factors

Failure to maintain a nothing-by-mouth status
Acute prostatitis

Nursing Implementation

• *Pretest*

Instruct the patient regarding the procedure and obtain written consent from the patient or person legally designated to make the patient's health care decisions.

Inform the patient to take a disposable phosphate (Fleet) enema on the night before or in the early morning. No food or fluids are permitted for 12 hours before the test since anesthesia is a possibility.

Assist the patient in removing all clothes and putting on a hospital gown.

Have the patient void to empty the bladder.

Place the patient in the lithotomy position.

• During the Test

For the transperineal approach, assist with the preparation of the local anesthetic. It will be injected by the physician into the perineal area between the scrotum and the rectum.

Provide comfort and reassurance to the patient who is anxious and afraid. Momentary pain is felt as the anesthetic is injected. Additionally, there is worry about the possible diagnosis.

Place the biopsy specimen in a sterile container with a preservative such as formalin or Zenker's fluid. In some cases, cultures or tissue slides are prepared immediately.

Label all specimens with the patient's name and the tissue source.

Send the specimens to the laboratory without delay.

Apply an adhesive bandage to the perineal biopsy site. No dressing is used for the transrectal approach.

• Posttest

Take vital signs and record the results. If general anesthesia was used or if the patient is unstable, continue monitoring the vital signs at regular intervals.

Assess for pain and offer pain medication as needed.

Observe the biopsy site for signs of bleeding on the dressing, or into local tissue.

Assess for difficulty in voiding or hematuria.

Instruct the patient to take the prescribed antibiotic to prevent infection.

✪ **COMPLICATION ALERT** ✪ Sepsis, bleeding, and perforation of the bladder or urethra are possible complications of a prostatic biopsy. The nurse should be aware that infection is most likely to occur in patients with a history of prostatitis or rheumatoid disorders.

PROSTATE-SPECIFIC ANTIGEN • SERUM

Synonym: PSA

N O R M A L   V A L U E S

Male
<39 years old: <2.0 ng/L
>39 years old: <2.8 ng/L

Purpose of the Test

In combination with the digital rectal examination, PSA is recommended as a screening tool for all men over the age of 50 years and for men over the age of 40 years who have additional risk factors, including African-American men and men who have a positive family history of prostate cancer. In addition, as a tumor marker for adenocarcinoma of the prostate gland, the PSA is used to monitor the postsurgical patient who has had a radical prostatectomy. It is used to evaluate for recurrence or residual tumor and helps identify the need for additional treatment.

Procedure

A red-topped tube is used to collect 1 ml of venous blood.

Findings

Increase

Adenocarcinoma of the prostate
Benign prostatic hypertrophy
Prostatitis
Urinary retention
Prostatic infarct

Interfering Factors

Recent urethral instrumentation

Nursing Implementation

- *Pretest*

Schedule the test at least 2 weeks after any urethral instrumentation procedure such as a transurethral resection, prostatic biopsy, or cystoscopy because these procedures will cause a release of the prostate-specific antigen.

Since a fasting specimen is preferred, instruct the patient to discontinue food intake for 8 hours before the test.

- *Posttest*

Arrange for prompt transport of the specimen to the laboratory.

✓ QUALITY CONTROL
Once the blood is centrifuged and the serum extracted, the serum is stable at room temperature for 24 hours. Thereafter, it must be stored at −20° C or less.

PROTEIN ELECTROPHORESIS • SERUM

NORMAL VALUES

Adult
  Albumin: 3.5–5.0 g/dL *or* SI 35–50 g/L
  Alpha$_1$-globulin: 0.1–0.3 g/dL *or* SI 1–3 g/L
  Alpha$_2$-globulin: 0.6–1.0 g/dL *or* SI 6–10 g/L
  Beta globulin: 0.7–1.1 g/dL *or* SI 7–11 g/L
  Gamma globulin: 0.8–1.6 g/dL *or* SI 8–16 g/L
Child
  Albumin: 3.6–5.2 g/dL *or* SI 36–52 g/L
  Alpha$_1$-globulin: 0.1–0.4 g/dL *or* SI 1–4 g/L
  Alpha$_2$-globulin: 0.5–1.2 g/dL *or* SI 5–12 g/L
  Beta globulin: 0.5–1.2 g/dL *or* SI 5–11 g/L
  Gamma globulin: 0.5–1.7 g/dL *or* SI 5–17 g/L

Purpose of the Test

Serum protein electrophoresis separates out and measures the amounts of the fractional protein components of the blood. The test is used in the detection of hepatobiliary disease, the evaluation of nutritional status, and the detection of multiple myeloma and macroglobulinemia.

Procedure

A red-topped sterile tube is used to collect 5 to 10 ml of venous blood.

Findings

Increase	*Decrease*
Albumin	*Albumin*
Dehydration	Rapid intravenous hydration
Alpha$_1$-globulin	Malnutrition
Inflammatory disease	Cirrhosis
Neoplastic disease	Cancer
Alpha$_2$-globulin	Nephrotic syndrome
Nephrotic syndrome	Crohn's disease
Neoplasm	Ulcerative colitis
Rheumatic fever	Severe thermal injury
Acute infection	Fistula
Beta globulin	*Alpha$_1$-globulin*
Hyperlipoprotenemia	Hereditary alpha$_1$-antitrypsin
Monoclonal gammopathies	deficiency
Gamma globulin	*Alpha$_2$-globulin*
Chronic liver diseases	Hemolysis
Collagen diseases	Hepatocellular damage
Infection	*Beta globulin*
Inflammation	Hypobetalipoproteinemia
Cancer	*Gamma globulin*
Myeloma	Response to cytoxic or immu-
Macroglobulinemia	nosuppressive medication
	Lymphocytic leukemia
	Lymphosarcoma
	Multiple myeloma
	Immunodeficiency syndrome

Interfering Factors

None

Nursing Implementation

• *Pretest*

No specific patient instruction or preparation is necessary.

PROTEIN ELECTROPHORESIS, 24-HOUR URINE	• URINE

Synonym: Urine protein electrophoresis

N O R M A L   V A L U E S

40–150 ng/24 hours *or* SI 40–150 mg/24 hours
No monoclonal gammopathy (M protein) noted

Purpose of the Test

Protein electrophoresis of the urine is used to identify the different types of protein loss in the urine and to evaluate patients with known or suspected multiple myeloma.

Procedure

A single voided specimen of urine is placed in a clean urine container.

Findings

Glomerular-Pattern Proteinuria

Glomerular diseases
Nephrotic syndrome

Tubular-Pattern Proteinuria

Falconi's syndrome
Cystinosis
Wilson's disease
Pyelonephritis
Renal transplant rejection

Overflow-Pattern Proteinuria

Multiple myeloma
Macroglobulinemia of Waldenströdom
Lymphoma
Amyloidosis

Interfering Factors

Hematuria

Nursing Implementation

- *Pretest*

Instruct the patient to collect a routine urine specimen.
Instruct female patients to collect the urine at a time when there is no menstrual flow.

- *Posttest*

Refrigerate the urine until it is transported to the laboratory.

PROTEINS • SERUM

N O R M A L   V A L U E S

TOTAL PROTEIN
Adult (ambulatory): 6.4–8.3 g/dL *or* SI 64–83 g/L
Child (>3 years): 6.0–8.0 g/dL *or* SI 60–80 g/L

ALBUMIN
Adult (18–60 years): 3.5–5.0 g/dL *or* SI 35–50 g/L
Child: 3.2–5.4 g/dL *or* SI 32–54 g/L

GLOBULIN: 2.8–4.4 g/dL *or* SI 28–44 g/L

ALBUMIN/GLOBULIN RATIO: >1

Purpose of the Tests

Total serum protein measurement provides a broad indicator of the quantity and concentration of all serum proteins except fibrinogen.

Serum albumin measurement is useful in the evaluation of nutritional status, oncotic pressure within the vasculature, and the effects of renal and other chronic diseases.

Globulin refers to the group of distinct globulin proteins. An abnormal value indicates the need for specific testing by serum protein electrophoresis.

The A/G ratio measures the proportion of the albumin and globulin components. A low A/G ratio demonstrates the severity and progression of the disease and indicates the need for specific additional data from serum protein electrophoresis.

Procedure

A red-topped sterile tube is used to collect 5 to 10 ml of venous blood. A capillary tube is used for newborns.

✓ QUALITY CONTROL
Venipuncture technique must be performed skillfully, since prolonged application of a tourniquet and hemolysis will give a false elevation of total protein value.

Findings

Increase

Total protein
Dehydration
Hyperimmunoglobulinemia
Polyclonal or monoclonal
    gammopathies
Albumin
Dehydration
Globulin
Inflammatory conditions
Multiple myeloma
Collagen diseases
Sarcoidosis
Cirrhosis
Chronic or active hepatitis

Decrease

Total protein
Crohn's disease
Ulcerative colitis
Intestinal fistula
Acute thermal injury
Nephrotic syndrome
Severe protein deficiency
Chronic liver disease
Malabsorption syndrome
Albumin
Rapid intravenous hydration
Malnutrition
Cirrhosis
Cancer
Nephrotic syndrome
Crohn's disease
Ulcerative colitis
Severe thermal injury
Gastrointestinal fistula
Collagen diseases
Infection and fever
Globulin
Agammaglobulinemia
Protein-losing enteropathies
Lymphomas
Multiple myeloma
A/G ratio
Cirrhosis
Chronic kidney disease
Sarcoidosis
Severe infection
Ulcerative colitis
Cachexia
Multiple myeloma
Severe thermal injury

Interfering Factors

Hemolysis
Prolonged bedrest
Massive intravenous infusion
Venous stasis
Peripheral vascular collapse
Hyperlipidemia
Hyperbilirubinemia

Nursing Implementation

• *Pretest*

If intravenous fluids are being administered, the blood sample is drawn from the opposite arm. This avoids local hemodilution and a false decrease in all protein values.

PROTHROMBIN TIME (PT, PROTIME)	• PLASMA

N O R M A L V A L U E S
Average: 10–13 seconds

Purpose of the Test

The prothrombin time is used to help screen for coagulation deficiency and to investigate the effects of liver failure and disseminated intravascular coagulation (DIC). It is also used to measure the response to oral coumarin (Coumadin) anticoagulant therapy.

In oral anticoagulant therapy, the therapeutic goal is a prothrombin time of 2 times the normal value. The possible panic value is 3 times more than the normal value.

The international normalized ratio (INR) provides a standardized measurement of the response to oral anticoagulant treatment. When the patient is adequately anticoagulated, the INR value should attain the therapeutic range of 2.0 to 3.0 for all conditions except for those with mechanical prosthetic heart valves. This condition requires an anticoagulant response that produces an INR of 2.5 to 3.5. With an INR >3.0, there is an increased risk of bleeding.

Procedure

A blue-topped tube with sodium citrate is used to obtain 4.5 ml of venous blood. As an alternative, a heelstick, earlobe, or finger puncture may be used to collect capillary blood in siliconized sodium citrate micropipettes.

✓ QUALITY CONTROL

The tube must be filled with blood. To mix the anticoagulant sodium citrate with the blood, the specimen tube is tilted gently from side to side 5 to 10 times.

When multiple samples are drawn, the PT specimen is obtained last. When this is the only test specimen, double-tube technique is used. A 1- to 2-ml blood sample is obtained and discarded and the blue-topped tube is then used to collect the test sample.

To prevent hemolysis, venipuncture technique must be smooth, with a blood flow that fills the vacuum tube readily.

Findings

Increase

Excess anticoagulant therapy
Deficiency of fibrinogen
Prothrombin
Factor V, VI, or X
Liver disease
Vitamin K deficiency
DIC

Interfering Factors

Lipemia
Hemolysis
Inadequate blood sample
Prolonged delay before analysis is performed

Nursing Implementation

• *Pretest*

Instruct the patient to discontinue intake of alcohol and caffeine for 24 hours before the test.
If the patient receives intermittent doses of heparin, ensure that the blood is drawn at least 2 hours after the last dose.

• *Posttest*

Ensure that the venipuncture site has sealed and that the patient is not bleeding. Use a sterile gauze to apply pressure to the puncture site as needed.

Arrange for prompt transport of the specimen to the laboratory. Any prothrombin time specimen received more than 2 hours after the blood is drawn is rejected.

PULMONARY FUNCTION STUDIES • SPIROMETRY

Synonyms: None

N O R M A L   V A L U E S

ADULT (70-KG MALE; 20–25% LOWER IN WOMEN)
Tidal volume (Vt): 500 ml
Inspiratory reserve volume (IRV): 3100 ml
Expiratory reserve volume (ERV): 1200 ml
Residual volume (RV): 1200 ml
Vital capacity (VC): 4800 ml
Inspiratory capacity (IC): 3600 ml
Functional residual capacity (FRC): 2400 ml
Total lung capacity (TLC): 6000 ml
FEV_1: 84%
FEV_2: 94%
FEV_3: 97%

Purpose of the Test

Pulmonary function studies are performed to evaluate the patient's respiratory status, especially in patients experiencing shortness of breath or other breathing difficulty. These studies may be used to evaluate the therapy for or progression of obstructive and restrictive lung disease. Portions of the test are used as parameters for weaning patients from mechanical ventilation and as part of preoperative evaluations.

A challenge or provocation test is included as part of the pulmonary function studies in patients with suspected hypersensitivities of the airways. *Bronchial provocation tests* or *bronchial challenge tests* are performed as part of the pulmonary function studies for patients who have symptoms suggestive of asthma but who do not show evidence of air flow limitations. They may also be used to assess airway function over time and to evaluate various therapeutic interventions. The provocation tests are contraindicated for anyone whose baseline Forced Expiratory Volume (FEV) is less than 1.5 L, who has a history of severe responses to identifiable antigens, or who has had a viral infection of the upper airway within 8 weeks prior to the test.

Procedure

Pulmonary function studies are usually performed in the respiratory therapy department or in a physician's office. To establish a closed system with the spirometer, a nose clip is placed over the patient's nose and the spirometer's mouthpiece is held in the mouth with the patient's lips maintaining an airtight seal. The patient is then instructed when to breathe normally, inhale maximally, and exhale maximally. This is repeated several times.

Findings

Increase

Functional residual capacity: Chronic obstructive pulmonary disease

Forced expiratory volume: Chronic obstructive pulmonary disease

Decrease

Tidal volume: Atelectasis, fatigue, pneumothorax, pulmonary congestion, restrictive lung disease, tumors

Inspiratory reserve volume: Asthma, exercise, obstructive pulmonary disease

Expiratory reserve volume: Ascites, kyphosis, obesity, pleural effusion, pneumothorax, pregnancy, scoliosis

Residual volume: Elderly individuals, obstructive pulmonary disease

Functional residual capacity: Adult respiratory distress syndrome

Forced expiratory volume: Restrictive pulmonary disease

Inspiratory capacity: Restrictive pulmonary disease

Vital capacity: Diaphragm restriction, drug overdose with hypoventilation, neuromuscular diseases, restrictive or depressed thoracic movement

Interfering Factors

Fatigue

Lack of patient cooperation

Smoking

Abdominal distention or pregnancy

Poor seal around mouthpiece (or tube)

Medications (analgesics, bronchodilators, sedatives)

Nursing Implementation

- *Pretest*

Assess the patient's cardiac status. Hold the test and notify the
physician if the patient has a history of angina or recent
myocardial infarction.

Maximize patient cooperation by explaining the procedure
and the need for full participation. Demonstrate the nose
clip and mouthpiece. The patient should wear dentures if
necessary for a proper mouth seal.

Instruct the patient not to smoke for 6 hours before the test.

Check with prescriber about administering bronchodilator and
intermittent positive-pressure breathing therapy before the
test.

Ensure that no constricting clothes are worn.

Ensure that oral intake is light to prevent stomach distention.

Instruct the patient to void immediately before the test.

Schedule the test before any other tests or procedures that
may fatigue the patient.

- *During the Test*

> ✓ QUALITY CONTROL
> If an abnormal response to a specific substance occurs during a
> provocation test, a placebo substance should be given to ensure
> that the bronchospasms were not induced by the spirometry.

- *Posttest*

Advise the patient to resume normal diet and activity.

Advise the patient to resume taking medications or receiving
therapy if held.

R

Synonyms: Kidney biopsy, fine needle aspiration biopsy of the kidney

N O R M A L   V A L U E S

Normal renal tissue is present, with no indication of inflammation, necrosis, or tumor cells

Purpose of the Test

Biopsy of the kidney provides specific information regarding the pathophysiologic changes in the tissue. The need for biopsy is determined on an individualized case basis. Other laboratory tests and noninvasive procedures are performed first to obtain as much diagnostic information as possible. The broad categories of pathophysiologic conditions that require renal biopsy include acute renal failure, renal tumor, renal transplant rejection, transplant failure, asymptomatic hematuria, proteinuria of unknown origin, or questions regarding drug toxicity and untoward reaction to medication. A renal biopsy may be done via a surgical incision (an open biopsy), which is rare or by fine needle biopsy (FNB).

Needle biopsy is often performed to diagnose renal cancer. It is used when computed tomography (CT) or magnetic resonance imaging (MRI) findings are inconclusive, to investigate metastatic disease or recurrence of cancer, and to diagnose the type of renal tumor in the patient who is a poor surgical risk. With fine needle aspiration biopsy, there is a small risk that the tumor will disseminate along the needle track.

In renal transplant patients, the donor kidney can show signs of transplant rejection. Without biopsy, early accurate diagnosis of rejection is difficult because of other possible causes of renal dysfunction that produce the same symptoms. Fine needle aspiration biopsy is minimally invasive and can be used repeatedly on the same patient.

Procedure

After administration of local anesthesia, a biopsy needle is inserted percutaneously or through a small incision in the lower back. While the needle is advanced into the kidney, ultrasound or x-ray films are used to guide the exact placement and location. A syringe is used to aspirate a small core of tissue from the renal cortex. The total time needed to obtain the specimen is about 15 minutes.

Findings

Acute or chronic glomerulonephritis
Goodpasture's syndrome
Amyloid infiltration of the kidney
Systemic lupus erythematosus
Renal transplant rejection or failure
Renal cell carcinoma
Wilms' tumor

Interfering Factors

Failure to maintain a nothing-by-mouth status
Coagulation disorders
Urinary tract infection
Nonfunction of one kidney

Nursing Implementation

• *Pretest*

Inform the patient about the procedure and obtain a written consent from the patient or person legally responsible for the patient's health care decisions.

Ensure that all screening tests are completed and that the results are posted in the patient's chart. Coagulation studies, including prothrombin time, activated partial thromboplastin time, platelet levels, and hematocrit, are performed to verify clotting ability. Urinalysis identifies the presence of any infection. An intravenous pyelogram or renal scan demonstrates renal function in both kidneys.

Take baseline vital signs and record the results.

• *During the Test*

Cleanse the skin of the lower back with antiseptic.

Provide reassurance to the patient to help alleviate anxiety.

When the needle is to be inserted, instruct the patient to take a deep breath and hold it. Assist the patient in remaining still. There may be brief pain, but it is mild.

✪ **COMPLICATION ALERT** ✪ Accidental perforation of the pleura during the FNB of the kidney may cause a pneumothorax. Assess patient for dyspnea, shortness of breath, cyanosis, restlessness, apprehension, and hypotension.

After the needle is removed, apply pressure to the puncture site for 20 minutes to help promote clotting.

Apply a sterile dressing and adhesive bandage to the puncture site.

Place the biopsy specimen in a sterile container with normal saline.

Ensure that the container is labeled with the patient's name and the tissue source of the specimen.

Arrange for immediate transport of the specimen to the laboratory.

✓ QUALITY CONTROL
On arrival at the laboratory, the specimen must be fresh and moist to ensure accurate analysis.

• *Posttest*

Take the vital signs every 15 minutes for 1 hour, every 30 minutes for the next hour, and at regular intervals thereafter.

At frequent intervals, observe the dressing and surrounding tissue for signs of bleeding.

For 8 hours, monitor each voided specimen for hematuria. Initially, a small amount of blood may be present, but it should disappear within the 8-hour period. In some institutions, the protocol is to collect every urine specimen separately, with a notation of the time and date of voiding written on the container. Over time, there should be progressively less blood, and the urine should return to its normal color.

Encourage the patient to drink extra fluids to help promote urination.

Eight hours after the test, ensure that a specimen for hemoglobin and hematocrit determinations is drawn. When bleeding is excessive, different time intervals and repeat testing may be necessary.

Instruct the patient to lie flat for 12 to 24 hours. A sandbag in the flank area may be used to help promote compression of the tissue. After this period of immobility, bedrest or limited activity is maintained for 24 hours to prevent the onset of fresh bleeding.

Instruct the patient to avoid physical exertion, heavy lifting, and trauma to the lower back for several days.

Assess for complications: Hematuria, infection, and perirenal hemorrhage.

RENIN • PLASMA

Synonym: Plasma renin activity, PRA

NORMAL VALUES

Recumbent position: 12–79 mU/L *or* SI 12–79 mU/L
Upright position: 13–114 mU/L *or* SI 13–114 mU/L

Purpose of the Test

Plasma renin levels are determined as part of hypertension screening and to diagnose primary aldosteronism.

Because renin is a powerful vasoconstrictor, its role in hypertension has been studied. Most patients with hypertension have normal renin levels. Some hypertensive patients with excessive fluid retention have low renin levels, and other hypertensive patients have high renin levels.

It has been difficult to correlate renin levels with clinical states, as renin levels vary between individuals and because laboratory techniques vary in the measurement of these levels. In addition, many factors will influence secretion rates of renin, including dietary ingestion of sodium. For this reason, some clinicians will correlate renin levels with the sodium content of the patient's diet. The sodium content of the diet is measured by a 24-hour urine sodium level.

Another method to evaluate renin is to perform a *sodium-*

depleted renin test, during which a diuretic (usually furosemide) is
given.

Procedure

Procedures vary. A random renin test simply requires a venipuncture to obtain 10 ml of blood in a lavender-topped tube containing EDTA. The specimen is placed on ice and immediately
sent to the laboratory. If the renin level is to be correlated with
sodium intake, a 24-hour urine specimen is required.

If a renin determination from a renal vein is planned, it is carried out under fluoroscopy; a catheter is inserted into the renal
vein via the femoral vein. The specimen is assayed by RIA.

Findings

Increase	*Decrease*
Hypertension	Fluid retention with high-sodium diet
Cirrhosis	
Hypovolemia	Primary aldosteronism
Hypokalemia	Excessive licorice intake
Addison's disease	Hypertension with fluid reten-tion
Chronic renal failure	
	Cushing's syndrome

Interfering Factors

Noncompliance with dietary and medication restrictions
Improper positioning during test
Medications (antihypertensives, clonidine, diuretics, estrogen,
  minoxidil, nitroprusside, propranolol, reserpine, vasodilators)

Nursing Implementation

The actions of the nurse vary depending on the technique used.

• *Pretest*

Instruct the patient on the technique.
If a random sampling is ordered, instruct the patient to maintain a prone position or an upright position for 2 hours before the test. The position is based on physician preference.
If a renal vein level is ordered, explain the need to go to the

radiology department for fluoroscopy. Explain equipment, groin preparation, and local anesthesia.

If a sodium depletion renin test is ordered, assess the patient's cardiovascular status before a diuretic is given.

Instruct the patient to maintain a low-sodium diet for 3 days before the test.

Check with the prescriber in regard to withholding interfering medications—for example, hypertensives, vasodilators, diuretics, or oral contraceptives—before the test.

• Posttest

If the femoral approach to the renal vein is used, assess the site for hematoma and bleeding.

☼ COMPLICATION ALERT ☼ Renin determination from a femoral vein access may cause bleeding or hematoma. Check *under* the patient for blood, as well as for other signs of bleeding. Observe and *palpate* over the access site for hematoma and check distal pulses, and temperature and color of involved extremity.

RESIN TRIIODOTHYRONINE UPTAKE	• SERUM

Synonyms: T_3 resin uptake test, RT_3U, T_3 uptake ratio

N O R M A L   V A L U E S

25–35% *or* SI 0.25–0.35
Free thyroxine index: 1.3–4.2
Free triiodothyronine index: 24–67

Purpose of the Test

The triiodothyronine resin uptake is determined to estimate the *free triiodothyronine index* and the *free thyroxine index*. In many institutions, the assay of free thyroid hormones has replaced the free triiodothyronine and thyroxine index because the indexes are estimates of the free hormone levels. The triiodothyronine resin uptake test is performed to diagnose hyper- and hypothyroidism.

Procedure

Venipuncture is performed to obtain a 10-ml serum specimen to which radioactive triiodothyronine is added. Radioactive triiodothyronine is used instead of thyroxine because more triiodothyronine is bound to the resin, as it has a lower affinity to endogenous protein-binding sites. After the resin is mixed with the radioactive triiodothyronine in serum, it is removed and the amount of radioactivity absorbed is measured.

The measurement of the free thyroxine and free triiodothyronine index is obtained by multiplying the resin uptake and the total thyroid hormone concentration. The indexes are not direct measurements of the free thyroid hormones, but estimates. However, the indexes do correlate with true free thyroid levels.

Findings

Increase	*Decrease*
Hyperthyroidism	Hypothyroidism

Interfering Factors

Renal failure
Malnutrition
Metastatic disease
Liver dysfunction
Critical illness
Medications (ACTH, androgens, barbiturates, chlorpromazine, estrogen, furosemide, glucocorticoids, heroin, lithium, methadone, phenylbutazone, propylthiouracil, thyroid replacement)

Nursing Implementation

The nurse takes actions similar to those taken in other venipuncture procedures.

RHEUMATOID FACTOR   •   SERUM, SYNOVIAL FLUID

Synonyms: RF, RA factor

NORMAL VALUES

Negative

Purpose of the Test

The test for rheumatoid factor is used in the diagnosis and prognosis of rheumatoid arthritis. Rheumatoid factor is present in the serum of the majority of patients with rheumatoid arthritis and other inflammatory conditions. Even though there is a high correlation between the presence of rheumatoid factor and rheumatoid arthritis, the exact nature of the relationship is unknown.

Procedure

A red-topped tube is used to collect 7 to 10 ml of venous blood.

Findings

Rheumatoid arthritis
Sjögren's syndrome
Systemic lupus erythematosus
Dermatomyositis
Scleroderma
Polymyositis
Waldenström's disease
Sarcoidosis
Infectious mononucleosis
Subacute bacterial endocarditis
Tuberculosis
Chronic lung disease
Chronic liver disease

Interfering Factors

Severe lipemia
Circulating immune complexes

Nursing Implementation

No special nursing measures are required.

S

NORMAL VALUES

Negative

Purpose of the Test

The sickle cell test is a screening test that is used to detect HbS, the sickling hemoglobin; to evaluate hemolytic anemia; and to help identify the cause of hereditary anemia.

Procedure

A lavender-topped tube is used to collect 7 ml of venous blood. As an alternative method, a fingerstick or earlobe puncture can be performed to obtain a capillary specimen, using lavender-topped micropipette tubes.

✓ QUALITY CONTROL
The tourniquet must not be applied tightly or for a prolonged time. To prevent hemolysis, the venipuncture should be smooth, with a blood flow that fills the tube readily.

Findings

Positive

Sickle cell anemia
Sickle cell trait
Other sickling disorders

Interfering Factors

Hemolysis
Coagulation of the specimen
Blood transfusion within the past 3 to 4 months

Nursing Implementation

• *Posttest*

Provide support to the parents who become upset when they learn of the abnormal findings. Additional testing must be performed to confirm the diagnosis.

SIGMOIDOSCOPY (PROCTOSCOPY) • ENDOSCOPY

N O R M A L   V A L U E S

No tissue abnormalities are seen.

Purpose of the Test

Sigmoidoscopy is used as a screening test for cancer of the colon. It is also used to investigate the source of unexplained rectal bleeding, to evaluate the postoperative anastomosis of the colon, and to diagnose or monitor inflammatory bowel disease.

Procedure

The patient is placed in a lateral or knee-chest (jackknife) position. Generally, no sedative anesthetic is needed. The well-lubricated instrument is inserted into the anus and advanced to the sigmoid colon. A tissue biopsy specimen, culture specimen, or sample of fecal matter may be obtained during the procedure.

Findings

Colitis
Colorectal cancer
"Gay bowel syndrome"
Crohn's disease
Irritable bowel syndrome
Sigmoid volvulus
Abscess
Intestinal ischemia
Parasitic disease
Adenomatous polyps

Interfering Factors

Uncooperative patient behavior
Severe bleeding

Suspected bowel perforation
Peritonitis
Toxic megacolon
Acute diverticulitis
Paralytic ileus

Nursing Implementation

- *Pretest*

Obtain a written consent.

Since bowel preparation varies among individuals, the examining physician should be consulted for specific instructions. The preparation usually consists of a combination of laxative and one or two Fleet enemas. The goal is to empty the lower colon of fecal matter.

- *During the Test*

Position and drape the patient.

Provide reassurance and promote relaxation during the procedure. A few deep breaths helps to relax the sphincter muscles.

Assist with the collection of tissue or other specimens.

- *Posttest*

Inform the patient that flatulence and mild gas pain may be experienced from the air that was put into the colon during the examination. When a biopsy is performed, it is normal to see a small amount of blood in the stool. Both of these effects are temporary.

Label the specimen container, including the name of the procedure and the tissue source. Send it to the laboratory without delay.

SIGNAL-AVERAGED ELECTROCARDIOGRAM	• ELECTROPHYSIOLOGY

Synonym: SAECG

N O R M A L   V A L U E S

Normal cardiac rhythm and conduction times

Purpose of the Test

Signal-averaged electrocardiography is a technique used to detect conduction defects that may precede ventricular tachycardia (VT). It is a noninvasive bedside test similar to a 12-lead ECG. With a signal-averaged ECG, the recording is obtained for 15 to 30 minutes, and the electric current from the heart is amplified 1000 times. The machine then integrates all these signals and removes extraneous electric signals.

The cardiologist assesses the printout of the signal-averaged ECG for late potentials, which place the patient at risk for sustained VT. A late potential is seen as a QRS complex that extends 20 to 60 msec into the ST segment.

Procedure

The procedure is similar to the 12-lead ECG, except that no limb electrodes are necessary and the six chest electrodes and ground lead are positioned differently on the chest.

Interfering Factors

Since the signal-averaged ECG averages the cardiac cycle of the patient, a relatively regular rhythm is needed during the test. *Frequent* premature atrial complexes or premature ventricular complexes interfere with the results. Signal-averaged electrocardiography is also unable to detect late potentials in patients with right or left bundle branch block.

Findings

Late potentials

Nursing Implementation

The nursing actions are similar to those for electrocardiography. In addition, review the following.

- *Pretest*

Check with the prescriber regarding discontinuing or administering the patient's antiarrhythmic medication.

- *During the Test*

Keep the environment quiet.
Instruct others to stay out of the patient's room.

SODIUM • SERUM

Synonym: Na+

NORMAL VALUES

Adult: 136–145 mEq/L *or* SI 136–145 μmol/L
Child: 138–145 mEq/L *or* SI 138–145 μmol/L
Infant: 139–146 mEq/L *or* SI 139–146 μmol/L
Newborn: 133–146 mEq/L *or* SI 133–146 μmol/L
Premature (48 hours): 128–148 mEq/L *or* SI 128–148 μmol/L

Purpose of the Test

Serum sodium levels are used to monitor electrolyte balance, water balance, and acid-base balance. They are also used in the evaluation of disorders of the central nervous system, musculoskeletal disorders, or diseases of the kidneys or adrenal glands. Serum sodium levels are part of the routine blood chemistry screen or SMA (sequential multiple analyzer).

Procedure

A red- or green-topped tube is used to obtain 5 to 7 ml of venous blood. For infants and small children, a heelstick, earlobe, or finger puncture and a capillary tube are used to obtain capillary blood.

✓ QUALITY CONTROL
Venipuncture technique must be smooth, with a blood flow that fills the tube readily. If the blood has excessive turbulence because of poor technique, the hemolysis of the erythrocytes will falsely elevate the test results.

Findings

Increase (hypernatremia)	*Decrease (hyponatremia)*
Dehydration	Addison's disease
Diabetic acidosis	Diuretic therapy
Cushing's syndrome	Hypopituitarism
Azotemia	Salt-wasting nephritis
Aldosteronism	Vomiting or diarrhea
Excessive saline infusion	Hypothyroidism
Profuse sweating	Burns

Increase (hypernatremia) (cont.)	*Decrease (hyponatremia) (cont.)*
Inadequate thirst	Glucocorticoid deficiency
Vomiting or diarrhea	Acute water intoxication
	Syndrome of inappropriate antidiuretic hormone
	Cirrhosis
	Acute or chronic renal failure
	Congestive heart failure
	Nephrotic syndrome
	Central nervous system disturbance (trauma, tumor)
	Ketonuria
	Bicarbonaturia

Interfering Factors

Hemolysis

Nursing Implementation

• *Pretest*

The blood should be drawn without a tourniquet to avoid clotting and hemolysis.

• *Posttest*

Arrange for prompt transport of the specimen to the laboratory.

> ✓ QUALITY CONTROL
> In the laboratory, the serum must be separated from the cells by centrifuge as soon as possible. This prevents clotting and hemolysis.

SPUTUM CULTURE AND SENSITIVITY (SPUTUM C & S) • SPUTUM

N O R M A L   V A L U E S

No growth

Purpose of the Test

These tests diagnose respiratory infections, identify the pathogenic organism responsible for the infection, and determine the appropriate antibiotic therapy.

Procedure

Expectoration Method. A sputum specimen may be obtained by the patient coughing up the sputum into a wide-mouthed sterile container with a cap.

Aspiration Method. When a bronchial specimen is needed, suctioning equipment and a sterile sputum trap are used to aspirate the specimen.

Bronchoscopy or Transtracheal Methods. A sputum specimen may be obtained during a bronchoscopy or via transtracheal aspiration. The nurse may assist with these procedures but does not perform them.

Findings

Positive

Pneumonia
Diphtheria
Influenza
Tuberculosis
Gonorrhea
Parasitic infection of the lungs

Interfering Factors

Contamination of the specimen
Antibiotic therapy

Nursing Implementation

- *Pretest*

Perform this test before antibiotic therapy is started.
Assess the patient's ability to follow instructions in coughing up the sputum as well as his or her ability to expectorate.
Plan to collect the specimen on arising in the morning before eating or drinking. Provide a sterile container with a cap.
Instruct the patient to take several deep breaths, cough up the

sputum from deep within the lungs, and expectorate into
the sterile container.

✓ QUALITY CONTROL

Demonstrate the procedure and have the patient perform a return demonstration to ensure that the container and lid are not
contaminated during the collection procedure. A major problem
with the expectoration method is contamination of the specimen by the microorganisms normally found in the mouth and
throat.

- *During the Test*

Expectoration Method

Support and encourage the patient's attempts to produce sputum. If it is not contraindicated, postural drainage, clapping,
and vibration may assist in raising the sputum. If the sputum
is very tenacious, aerosol therapy may be necessary.

Approximately 1 tsp. of sputum is necessary for this test. When
the patient is unable to produce this amount in one at-
tempt, the container should be capped between attempts to
expectorate.

Aspiration Method

If the patient is entubated, a sputum trap is used to aspirate the
specimen. The sputum trap is inserted between the sterile suction catheter and the suction tubing attached to the wall suction
regulator. The patient is suctioned by the usual method. To use
the sputum trap:

1. Tighten the cap to obtain an airtight seal.
2. Attach the wall suction tubing to the plastic "chimney" on
   the cap.
3. Connect the distal end of the sterile container to the latex
   tubing.
4. Suction as usual, but do not flush the catheter while the trap
   is in place.
5. After suctioning, disconnect the suction tubing and catheter.
6. Connect the latex tubing to the "chimney" of the cap.

- *Posttest*

Ensure that the container is tightly sealed and correctly labeled. Send the specimen to the laboratory as soon as possible. Do not refrigerate the specimen.

⊘ **COMPLICATION ALERT** ⊘ There are no specific complications in obtaining a sputum culture and sensitivity test. The nurse should be aware of the complications of endotracheal suctioning, however, if the aspiration method is used to obtain the specimen.

| STRESS TESTING, CARDIAC | • ELECTROPHYSIOLOGY |

Synonyms: Graded exercise testing (GEX), graded exercise stress testing (GEST), exercise stress testing, exercise electrocardiography

NORMAL VALUES

No unexpected changes in the ECG

Purpose of the Test

Stress testing is an important noninvasive procedure for evaluating the cardiovascular status of patients who are known to have cardiac disease or who are at risk for cardiac disease. The test increases the demand placed on the heart by increasing physical activity. Through electrocardiographic tracings, it can be determined whether the heart is able to meet the increased oxygen demand. Stress testing is an invaluable technique in (1) assessing the at-risk population, (2) diagnosing chest pain syndromes and dysrhythmias associated with ischemia, (3) evaluating the effectiveness of therapy (surgical or pharmacologic), and (4) identifying the initial level of function in cardiac rehabilitation programs and evaluating the results.

Procedure

Exercise stress testing requires the use of a bicycle ergometer or a treadmill with continuous electrocardiac recording. The test is performed in a series of stages in which the patient exercises for 3 minutes. At the end of each stage, a 12-lead ECG is recorded. After each stage, the workload or "graded load" is increased. This is accomplished by increasing the speed or resistance of the bicycle or treadmill. The stress testing continues until the patient reaches the maximum heart rate, becomes symptomatic, or displays electrocardiographic changes consistent with ischemia. The maximum heart rate is usually determined by normograms. A gross estimate of the maximum heart rate is 220 beats per minute minus the patient's age.

If a patient is physically unable to exercise to the point of maximum heart rate, a *pharmacologic stress test* may be done with *dipyridamole (Persantine)*. Many patients who are candidates for stress testing are not able to perform the exercise required because of peripheral vascular disease or pulmonary, orthopedic, or neurologic dysfunction. Dipyridamole may be given intravenously or by mouth. It causes coronary artery dilation similar to the response of the coronary arteries to exercise. After peak effect is reached (85% maximum heart rate), a thallium scan may be performed (see pp. 301–302). A follow-up scan is performed 4 hours later.

Findings

A 1-mm depression of the ST segment is a positive stress test, indicating myocardial ischemia.

Interfering Factors

Severe anxiety may interfere with the patient's ability to participate fully in the stress testing. False-positive results may be due to bundle branch block, ventricular hypertrophy, or digitalization. False-negative results may be due to the use of beta-blockers.

Nursing Implementation

- *Pretest*

Instruct the patient about the purpose and procedure of the test.

Inform the patient to wear comfortable clothes and rubber-soled walking shoes.

Instruct the patient not to eat, smoke, or drink alcohol for 3 to 4 hours before the test.

Assess for contraindications to stress testing: Chest pain, unstable angina with recent chest pain, uncontrolled hypertension, acute myocarditis or pericarditis, thrombophlebitis, second- or third-degree heart block, serious dysrhythmias, severe congestive heart failure, severe hypertrophic obstructive cardiomyopathy, neurologic, musculoskeletal, or vascular problems that would impede mobility on the bicycle or treadmill.

• *During the Test*

Have emergency equipment and drugs available (code cart).
The patient is attached to electrodes for recording a 12-lead ECG.
A blood pressure cuff is put in place for quick access. A baseline blood pressure reading is obtained.
As the graded exercises begin, a multichanneled ECG is recorded. A 12-lead ECG is recorded and the blood pressure is checked as each workload ends (every 3-minute increment).
Observe for signs to stop the stress testing, for example, falling blood pressure, three consecutive premature ventricular contractures, chest pain, severe dyspnea, or exhaustion. The stressing may or may not be discontinued if ST depressions occur, blood pressure does not rise, or frequent or coupled premature ventricular contractions or bundle branch block occurs.
If dipyridamole was used, assess for side effects: myocardial infarction, dysrhythmias, bronchospasms, chest pain, nausea, headache, flushing hypotension, and dizziness.

✪ **COMPLICATION ALERT** ✪ During the stress test, the nurse continuously assesses the patient for indications of myocardial ischemia. Communicate with patients so they will be free to report chest pain. Continuously observe the cardiac monitor for dysrhythmias and ST elevations or depressions.

• *Posttest*

Cardiac monitoring is continued for 5 to 10 minutes after the testing to evaluate the patient's physiologic response.
Blood pressure is checked.
Remove conduction jelly and assist in robing the patient if necessary.
Evaluate the patient's physical and emotional response to the testing.
Instruct the patient to rest and not to take hot showers or baths for 2 to 4 hours.

SYPHILIS SEROLOGY   •   SERUM

N O R M A L   V A L U E S

Venereal disease research laboratory (VDRL): Nonreactive
Rapid plasma reagin (RPR): Nonreactive
Automated reagin test (ART): Nonreactive
Fluorescent treponemal antibody absorption (FTA-ABS):
Nonreactive
Microhemagglutin *Treponema pallidum* (MHA-TP):
Nonreactive

Purpose of the Tests

The VDRL, RPR, and ART are used to screen for syphilis. Because of the possibility of a false positive test result, the FTA-ABS and the MHA-TP are used to confirm the diagnosis of syphilis. The VDRL test is used to monitor the response to therapy.

Procedure

A red-topped tube is used to collect 7 ml of venous blood.

✓ QUALITY CONTROL
The tourniquet should be tied lightly for a brief time to prevent pooling of cells in the vein at the site of blood collection. To prevent hemolysis, venipuncture technique must be smooth, with a blood flow that fills the vacuum tube readily.

Findings

Positive

Syphilis

Interfering Factors

Lipemia
Alcohol
Hemolysis

Nursing Implementation

Pretest

Instruct the patient to avoid alcohol intake for 24 hours before the test. Fasting for 8 hours is also recommended to reduce the serum lipid content.

- *Posttest*

Arrange for prompt transport of the specimen to the laboratory. The MHA-TP specimen requires refrigeration when
there is a delay before analysis can be performed.

Instruct the patient to abstain from sexual contact until the results are known. If the result is positive, abstinence continues until the infection is treated and cured. The patient
should inform all sexual partners of the test results. Sexual
contacts are advised to undergo testing.

Positive test results are reported to the state health department.

T

TESTOSTERONE, TOTAL, FREE • SERUM

NORMAL VALUES

TOTAL TESTOSTERONE
Adult male: 300–1000 ng/dl *or* SI 10.4–34.7 nmol/L
Adult female: 20–75 ng/dl *or* SI 0.69–2.6 nmol/L
Child (1–10 years): <3–10 ng/dl *or* SI <0.1–0.35 nmol/L

FREE TESTOSTERONE
Adult male: 52–280 pg/ml *or* SI 180.4–971.6 pmol/L
Adult female: 1.6–6.3 pg/ml *or* SI 5.6–21.9 pmol/L
Child (1–10 years): 0.15–0.66 pg/ml *or* SI 0.5–2.1 pmol/L

Purpose of the Test

These tests are used to diagnose precocious sexual development, deficient activity of the testes or ovaries, male infertility or sexual dysfunction, and female virilization.

Procedure

A red-topped tube is used to collect 7 ml of venous blood.

Findings

Increase	*Decrease*
Tumor (ovary, adrenal, testicle)	Cirrhosis
	Hypopituitarism
Central nervous system lesion	Estrogen therapy
Hyperthyroidism	Severe obesity
Congenital adrenal hyperplasia	Renal failure
	Malnutrition
Idiopathic precocious puberty	Cryptorchidism

Interfering Factors

Recent radioactive isotope scan

Nursing Implementation

- *Pretest*

Schedule this test before or at least 7 days after a nuclear scan.

| **THALLIUM TESTING** | • RADIONUCLIDE IMAGING |

Synonyms: Thallium scan, thallium exercise imaging, resting thallium scan

N O R M A L   V A L U E S

Normal myocardial perfusion; no "cold spots"

Purpose of the Test

Thallium is a radioactive analog of potassium, which is rapidly taken up by myocardial cells. After thallium-201 is given, almost 90% of it is extracted by the myocardium within seconds. For this to occur, two factors are essential: (1) adequate perfusion and (2) cellular extraction efficiency. Since cellular ischemia does not seem to affect thallium uptake in the myocardium, its lack of uptake is an indication of an infarction.

Thallium imaging is used to assess coronary blood flow to determine areas of infarction and ischemia. It is used to diagnose CAD and assess revascularization following coronary artery bypass surgery.

Procedure

Thallium scanning is performed with an Anger gamma camera combined with a computer. Continuous counts of emitted photons are made during the cardiac cycle. The scan identifies "cold spots," areas of decreased thallium uptake. "Cold spots" identify areas of ischemia and infarction. Thallium can be given under a state of no physical demand, which is known as a *resting thallium study,* or it can be part of a stress test, in which case it is called *exercise thallium imaging.* Exercise thallium imaging distinguishes ischemic sites from infarcted areas. Thallium scans are repeated, once during stress testing and then 3 to 4 hours after the thallium was given and the stress test was completed. With the second imaging, if a "cold spot" remains, it is assumed to be an infarcted area. If the "cold spot" disappears, it is recognized as an ischemic area.

For patients who cannot perform an exercise stress test, adenoscan (adenosine) may be used to pharmacologically stress the heart.

Findings

Cold spots indicate and distinguish areas of infarction and ischemia.

Interfering Factors

See discussion of stress testing.

Nursing Implementation

Nursing care is similar to that in stress testing, except that the patient has an infusion of normal saline started.

- *Pretest*

Usually, long-acting nitrates are held for 8 to 12 hours before the test.

If adenoscan is used, check for contraindications: Hypersensitivity to adenoscan, sinus node disease, second or third degree A-V block, asthma or other bronchospasmic disorder, acute myocardial infarction, and hypotension.

- *During the Test*

The thallium is given intravenously about a minute before the completion of the stress test.

After the completion of the stress test, the patient is placed supine on the table, and multiple scintigraphic images are taken.

- *Posttest*

Assess the patient's response.

Three to four hours later, the patient returns for repeat films.

THORACENTESIS • PATHOLOGY

Synonyms: Pleural fluid analysis, pleural tap

N O R M A L V A L U E S
Normal pleural fluid
No pathogens or malignant cells

Purpose of the Test

Thoracentesis is performed to remove fluid from the pleural space for diagnostic or therapeutic reasons. Pleural effusions (accumulation of fluid in the pleural space) may be due to neoplastic or infectious processes or leakage of fluid from the vascular system. If the effusion is due to neoplasms or infection, the fluid is usually called an exudate. If the fluid is due to leakage from the blood vessels, it is called transudate. To distinguish between exudates and transudates, pleural fluid is evaluated for protein, specific gravity, and glucose, and a blood cell count with differential is performed.

Pleural fluid is also obtained for cultures to identify tuberculosis, fungal and various bacterial infections. Cytologic examination of the pleural fluid is performed to rule out malignancy.

Procedure

After the patient is positioned in a seated, upright position, the lower posterior chest is exposed and prepared, and a local anesthetic is given. A needle is inserted into the pleural space. The fluid is aspirated. A pleural biopsy may be performed at this time.

If a *pleural biopsy* is planned, a special biopsy needle with a hooked biopsy trocar is used. Usually three specimens are obtained from three pleural sites. Specimens are placed in fixative and sent to the laboratory immediately.

Findings

Bacterial, viral, or fungal infection
Malignancy
Collagen disease
Lymphoma
Systemic lupus erythematosus
Liver failure
Nephrotic syndrome
Myxedema
Pancreatitis

Interfering Factors

Uncooperative patient

Nursing Implementation

• *Pretest*

Explain the procedure and the purpose of the test to the patient.

Ensure that a signed consent form has been obtained.

Perform and document a baseline assessment. A blood pressure cuff is left in place to permit easy monitoring of the blood pressure during the procedure.

Initiate supplemental O_2 if ordered.

Check the PT, PTT, and platelet count to identify potential bleeding problems.

Instruct the patient not to cough or move during the procedure.

Obtain a thoracentesis tray from supply room.

• During the Test

Continuously monitor the patient's response to the procedure.

Observe the pulse oximeter, if in use, for changes in Svo_2.

Position the patient in an upright position, seated on the side of the bed with the legs resting on a footstool. The patient's arms should be supported on a padded overbed table. If the patient is unable to sit up, he or she may lie on the unaffected side, with the back flush with the edge of the bed.

Provide emotional support to the patient, as pressure pain may be experienced even though local anesthesia is given.

After the needle is inserted with a stopcock attached, fluid is drawn off for analysis. A catheter may be inserted at this point if a large amount of fluid is to be drained.

When a biopsy is performed, instruct the patient to exhale fully and perform the Valsalva maneuver to prevent air from entering the pleural space when the tissue sample is taken.

• Posttest

Check vital signs every 15 minutes until they are stable.

Assess for bilateral breath sounds.

Document amount, color, and character of the fluid obtained.

Obtain a chest radiograph as ordered to check for pneumothorax.

Encourage the patient to lie on the uninvolved side for 1 hour to improve oxygenation.

Check small dressing over the site for bleeding or drainage. Palpate around the site for subcutaneous emphysema.

Assess patient for pneumothorax, bleeding, and infection.

⊗ **COMPLICATION ALERT** ⊗ While the major complication following thoracentesis is pneumothorax, the nurse needs to assess for another serious complication, *reexpansion pulmonary edema*. It occurs if large amounts of pleural fluid are removed, which causes an increase in negative intrapleural pressure. If the lungs do not reexpand to fill the space, edema can result.

THYROID BIOPSY • PATHOLOGY

Synonyms: None

NORMAL VALUES

Normal cells

Purpose of the Test

A biopsy is performed to differentiate the cause of thyroid nodules or lumps. Thyroid nodules are more common in women and occur at any age. Thyroid cancer is rare; most nodules are benign. The biopsy will identify malignant thyroid nodules, follicular neoplasms, and benign lesions.

Procedure

A thyroid biopsy is usually performed by fine needle aspiration (FNA). FNA has replaced surgical removal as a diagnostic technique because it avoids surgical risk and is less traumatic for the patient. FNA is usually carried out in the operating room to maintain sterile technique. It usually requires a local anesthetic only, which permits it to be performed on an outpatient basis. A 23- or 25-gauge biopsy needle is used to aspirate tissue from the nodule. The tissue is assessed by cytologic examination.

Findings

Benign thyroid nodules
Cancer of the thyroid gland
Follicular neoplasm (cancerous or benign)

Interfering Factors

Noncompliance with dietary restrictions
Failure to place specimen in preservative immediately after aspiration
Inadequate amount of tissue obtained

Nursing Implementation

• *Pretest*

Assess the patient's level of anxiety, as fear of cancer may be significant or may interfere with the patient's ability to understand explanations.

Instruct the patient not to eat or drink for 12 hours before the test.

Prepare the patient for the operating room according to hospital protocol.

Ensure that a signed informed consent form has been obtained.

Administer preprocedure medication as prescribed.

• *During the Test*

The patient is positioned on the back with a small pillow under the shoulders.

Usually, a local anesthetic is given. General anesthesia may be required in some cases.

Encourage the patient not to move or swallow as the local anesthetic is being given.

Support the patient, who will feel pressure as the procedure is performed.

• *Posttest*

Reassure the patient that tenderness at the biopsy site is normal.

Position the patient in a semi-Fowler's position with a small pillow under the head to remove stress from the site.

Instruct the patient to support the head when changing position.

Keep site clean and dry.

Observe for bleeding, edema, and infection.

✪ **COMPLICATION ALERT** ✪ Covert bleeding following a thyroid biopsy may cause hematoma formation. The nurse must observe the site, check for dyspnea, and listen for a stridor.

THYROTROPIN • SERUM

Synonyms: Thyroid-stimulating hormone, TSH

N O R M A L   V A L U E S

Adult: 0.4–8.9 U/ml *or* SI 0.4–8.9 mU/L
Newborn, whole blood: <20 U/ml *or* SI <20mU/L

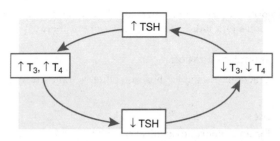

Figure 6. Thyroid Hormone Regulation. Thyroid hormone production and secretion is based on a negative feedback mechanism with thyroid-stimulating hormone (TSH) secreted by the anterior pituitary gland.

Purpose of the Test

Thyrotropin is secreted by the anterior pituitary gland via a negative feedback mechanism (see Fig. 6). Thyrotropin causes the thyroid gland to increase its production and secretion of thyroid hormones.

Thyrotropin levels are obtained to (1) diagnose hypothyroidism, (2) distinguish between primary and secondary hypothyroidism, and (3) monitor patient response to thyroid replacement therapy.

Procedure

Venipuncture is performed to obtain 7 ml of blood in a red-topped tube. If the test is required on a newborn, a heelstick is performed and the blood is collected on filter paper.

Findings

Increase	*Decrease*
Addison's disease	Hyperthyroidism
Goiter (some forms)	Overdose of exogenous thy-
Hyperpituitarism	roid replacement
Pituitary adenoma	Secondary hypothyroidism
Primary hypothyroidism	Tertiary hypothyroidism
Thyroid cancer	Thyroiditis

Interfering Factors

Radioisotope administration within 1 week
Extreme stress

Medications (aspirin, corticosteroids, dopamine, heparin, lithium, potassium iodide, thyroid replacement therapy)

Nursing Implementation

Nursing actions resemble those of other venipuncture procedures.

• *Pretest*

Assess for and report any clinical states that would increase the patient's endogenous glucocorticoid levels.

Check with prescriber regarding withholding medications that may interfere with test results.

THYROXINE   • SERUM

Synonym: T$_4$

N O R M A L   V A L U E S

Adult: 5–12 µg/dl *or* SI 64.4–154.4 nmol/L
Children
  10–20 years: 4.2–11.8 µg/dl *or* SI 54.11–151.9 nmol/L
  1–10 years: 6.4–15 µg/dl *or* SI 82.41–193.1 nmol/L
  2–10 months: 7.8–16.5 µg/dl *or* SI 100.4–212.4 nmol/L
Newborn: 6.4–23.2 µg/dl *or* SI 82.4–298.6 nmol/L

Purpose of the Test

Thyroxine levels are obtained to evaluate thyroid function, confirm the diagnosis of hyper- or hypothyroidism, and evaluate therapy for hyper- or hypothyroidism.

Procedure

Venipuncture is performed to obtain 5 ml of blood in a red-topped tube. RIA is used to assess the hormone level.

If a thyroxine determination is ordered on a newborn, umbilical cord blood may be used *or* a heelstick can be performed. With the heelstick method, special filter paper is used to blot the blood, and the filter paper is sent to the laboratory in a container that protects against light.

Findings

Increase	*Decrease*
Hyperthyroidism	Hypothyroidism
Acute or subacute thyroiditis	Chronic or subacute thyroiditis
	Myxedema
	Cretinism

Interfering Factors

Liver disorders (which affect blood protein levels)

Protein-wasting diseases such as chronic renal failure

Medications (androgens, aspirin, chlorpropamide, chlorpromazine, estrogen, heparin, iodides, thyroid replacement medications, lithium, methadone, phenothiazines, phenytoin, reserpine, steroids, sulfonamides, sulfonylureas, tolbutamide)

Nursing Implementation

Nursing actions are similar to those used in other venipuncture procedures.

• During the Test

If a heelstick is performed, the heel is first cleansed with antiseptic and the skin is pierced with a sterile lancet. Completely saturate the circles on the filter paper.

Since pregnancy will normally cause an increase in thyroxine levels, indicate on the requisition slip if the patient is pregnant.

• Posttest

Send filter paper to the laboratory in a container that protects against light.

THYROXINE-BINDING GLOBULIN	• SERUM

Synonym: TBG

NORMAL VALUES

16–34 µg/ml *or* SI 16–34 mg/L

Purpose of the Test

Thyroxine-binding globulin (TBG) is the primary protein carrier of thyroxine and triiodothyronine. The thyroid hormones bound to TBG provide a storehouse of the hormones, which are released from the protein as needed. Since TBG carries approximately 70% of the total amount of thyroid hormones in the circulation, TBG levels significantly affect total hormone concentrations. TBG is evaluated when clinical manifestations of thyroid dysfunction and thyroid hormone levels do not correlate.

Procedure

Venipuncture is performed to collect 7 ml of blood in a red-topped tube. TBG levels are assessed by RIA or electrophoresis.

Findings

Increase	*Decrease*
Congenital abnormality	Androgens
Estrogen therapy	Cirrhosis of the liver
Acute hepatitis	Congenital abnormality
Hypothyroidism	Glucocorticoids
Pregnancy	Hyperthyroidism
	Recent surgery
	Renal failure
	Starvation

Interfering Factor

Heparin
Phenylbutazone
Phenytoin
Salicylates

Nursing Implementation

The nurse takes actions similar to those taken in other venipuncture procedures.

- *Pretest*

Obtain a medication history to determine if any drug is being taken that affects normal thyroid binding.

TOXOPLASMOSIS SEROLOGY • SERUM

NORMAL VALUES

IgM antibody titer: <1:8

Purpose of the Test

This test helps to diagnose toxoplasmosis. It identifies antibody formation that results from exposure to the sporozoan parasite.

Procedure

A red-topped tube is used to collect 7 ml of venous blood.

Findings

Increase

Toxoplasmosis

Interfering Factors

None

Nursing Implementation

- *Pretest*

Schedule the test to be performed at the onset of illness and 2 to 3 weeks later during the convalescent phase.

TRIIODOTHYRONINE • SERUM

Synonym: T_3

NORMAL VALUES
Adult: 40–204 ng/dl *or* SI 0.6–3.1 nmol/L
Children
10–20 years: 80–213 ng/dl *or* SI 1.2–3.3 nmol/L
1–10 years: 105–269 ng/dl *or* SI 1.6–4.1 nmol/L
1–12 months: 105–245 ng/dl *or* SI 1.6–3.7 nmol/L
Newborn: 100–740 ng/dl *or* SI 1.5–11.4 nmol/L

Purpose of the Test

Triiodothyronine levels are obtained as part of the diagnostic process to determine hyper- or hypothyroidism and to diagnose triiodothyronine toxicosis.

Procedure

Venipuncture is performed to obtain 3 ml of blood in a red-topped tube.

Findings

Increase

Hyperthyroidism
Pregnancy
Toxic adenoma of the thyroid gland
Toxic nodular goiter

Decrease

Hypothyroidism
Liver disease
Recent surgery
Renal disease

Interfering Factors

Significant increase or decrease in thyroxine-binding globulins
Medications (estrogen, heparin, iodides, triiodothyronine replacement therapy, lithium, methadone, methimazole, methylthiouracil, phenylbutazone, phenytoin, progestins, propranolol, propylthiouracil, reserpine, salicylates, steroids, sulfonamides)

Nursing Implementation

Nursing actions are similar to those for other venipuncture procedures.

TROPONIN • SERUM

Synonyms: Cardiac Troponin T, cT$_n$T, cardiac Troponin I, cT$_n$I

N O R M A L   V A L U E S

Cardiac Troponin T: <0.2 µg/L *or* SI <0.2 µg/L
Cardiac Troponin I: <3.1 µg/L *or* SI <3.1 µg/L

Purpose of the Test

Troponin T is a protein found in skeletal and cardiac muscle fibers. Troponin I is a protein found in cardiac muscle complex; therefore, it is very specific to the heart. Troponin levels increase earlier than CK-MB; therefore, they may be helpful in diagnosing myocardial infarction earlier than traditional cardiac enzyme studies. Earlier diagnosis may lead to earlier thrombolytic therapy.

Procedure

A venipuncture is performed to obtain 5 ml of blood in a red-topped tube.

Findings

Increase in Troponin T & I
Acute myocardial infarction

Increase in Troponin T
Renal failure
Muscle trauma
Rhabdomylitis
Polymyositis
Dermatomyositis

Interfering Factors

Hemolysis of specimen

✓ QUALITY CONTROL
Troponin T may increase in patients with angina; therefore, it is not specific for an acute myocardial infarction for patients with chest pain.

Nursing Implementation

Similar to other venipunctures. Ensure specimen is drawn on admission or on the occurrence of chest pain and then at 4, 8, 12, and 24 hours.

TYPE AND CROSSMATCH (COMPATIBILITY TEST)	• BLOOD

N O R M A L   V A L U E S
Not applicable

Purpose of the Test

Human blood is typed by group, based on the presence or absence of A, B, AB, O, and Rh antigens. In preparation for transfusion, type and crossmatching tests are performed to determine the major blood groups, and to determine the compatibility of the blood of the recipient and the potential donor. The indirect antiglobulin test is also done to screen for antibodies. In selecting a donor's blood that matches that of the recipient, there must be a compatibility of antigens and antibodies so that the transfusion is safe for the recipient.

Procedure

Two red-topped tubes and a lavender-topped tube are used to collect 7 ml of venous blood in each tube.

✓ QUALITY CONTROL
To prevent hemolysis of the erythrocytes, the tourniquet must be tied lightly and for a brief time only. Venipuncture technique must be smooth, with a blood flow that fills the vacuum tube readily.

Findings

Positive

In the crossmatch of donor and recipient blood, there is incompatibility.

Negative

In the crossmatch of donor and recipient blood, there is probable compatibility.

Interfering Factors

Hemolysis
Inadequate identification procedure

Nursing Implementation

• *Pretest*

When blood is to be drawn, the intended recipient must be identified with absolute certainty by the person who draws the blood:

1. The intended recipient must state his or her name.
2. The hospital wristband is compared with the verbal identification.

A transfusion wristband is applied to the recipient's wrist. This wristband contains the recipient's name, hospital identification number, and the date and initials of the phlebotomist.

The specimen tubes and the requisition form are also labeled with the same identification information.

The requisition form is signed by the phlebotomist, indicating that all identification information has been verified on the two wristbands and by the intended recipient.

• *Posttest*

Once the type and crossmatch is completed, the donor blood units are available for the recipient. Donor crossmatched blood is usually held for no more than 24 hours.

Use the same, careful identification procedure when the blood is to be administered. The consequences of an error in identification are profound and can result in the death of the patient.

U

ULTRASOUND (SONOGRAM) • SOUNDWAVE IMAGING

N O R M A L   V A L U E S

There are no anatomic or functional abnormalities. The organs are normal in size, shape, contour, and position. The internal structures of the organs and tissues are within normal limits.

Purpose of the Test

Ultrasound examines organs, blood vessels, and structures of the body to identify malposition, malformation, malfunction, or abnormal tissue growth. It is also used to provide visualization during an invasive procedure such as biopsy or needle aspiration.

Procedure

High-frequency sound waves are directed into an area of the body in a specific pattern. The echoes of the ultrasound are converted to visual images, linear tracings, or audible sounds.

Findings

Tumor
Cyst
Hypertrophy
Vascular occlusion
Atherosclerotic plaque
Venous thrombosis
Obstruction or stricture
Abscess
Calculus
Congenital anomaly
Aneurysm
Hematoma
Bleeding

Foreign body
Pregnancy
Fetal development

Interfering Factors

Air
Bowel gas
Overlying bones
Barium
Obesity

Nursing Implementation

- *Pretest*

No consent is needed for the routine ultrasound examination
that uses an external transducer and a noninvasive method
of examination.

Schedule the ultrasound examination before or several days
after any barium studies.

✓ QUALITY CONTROL
Barium is an opaque substance that blocks the transmission of
ultrasound impulses. Residual barium causes an ultrasound problem for about 24 hours after a barium x-ray examination.

Instruct the patient about any dietary restrictions or modifications. Any abdominal ultrasound examination requires fasting from food for 12 hours. If the patient has a tendency toward bowel gas, a low-residue diet is implemented for 24 to
36 hours, followed by a 12-hour fast from all foods. Some abdominal ultrasound protocols require an enema before the
examination. Schedule the abdominal tests for the early
morning. Gynecologic ultrasound procedures often require
drinking 40 oz. of water without voiding before the test.
This fills the urinary bladder and moves it upward and away
from the uterus.

✓ QUALITY CONTROL
Intestinal gas must be removed from the colon because ultrasound impulses cannot pass through air.

Inform the patient that the examination is safe and painless. A small child or agitated, anxious patient may be accompanied by a calming parent or adult.

Assist the patient in removing all clothes, jewelry, and metallic objects. A hospital gown is worn.

• *During the Test*

Position the patient on the examining table.

Instruct the patient to remain still during the examination.

Apply the acoustic gel to the skin surface in the area to be examined. The gel serves as a conducting agent and eliminates the thin layer of air that would block the transmission of impulses.

• *Posttest*

Remove the acoustic gel to prevent the soiling of the patient's clothes.

UPPER GASTROINTESTINAL AND SMALL BOWEL SERIES   • RADIOLOGY

NORMAL VALUES

No structural or functional abnormalities are found.

Purpose of the Test

The upper GI series detects disorders of structure or function of the esophagus, stomach, and duodenum. It may also be used to evaluate the results of gastric surgery. If it is done, the small bowel series detects disorders of the jejunum or ileum.

Procedure

The patient drinks a barium solution to provide viewing of swallowing and peristalsis in the esophagus. As the barium coats the mucosal lining of the stomach, x-rays are taken to outline the shape and contour of that organ. For a small bowel series, fluoroscopy demonstrates the passage of the barium through the intestine. Radiographic films document any abnormality.

Findings

Esophagus

Foreign body
Neuromuscular incoordination or weakness
Stricture
Spasm
Hiatal hernia
Polyps
Tumor
Cancer
Ulcers
Esophagitis
Varices

Stomach

Peptic ulcer
Cancer
Pyloric obstruction
Benign tumor
Inflammatory disease
Perforation
Diverticula

Small Bowel

Malabsorption
Crohn's disease
Hodgkin's disease
Lymphosarcoma
Diffuse sclerosis
Perforation
Intussusception

Interfering Factors

Failure to maintain the nothing-by-mouth status
Excess air in the small bowel

Nursing Implementation

- *Pretest*

Explain the procedure to the patient and obtain a written consent.

Instruct the patient to fast from all food for 8 hours and all liquids for 4 hours before the test.

Most oral medications are withheld in the 8 hours before the test. Narcotics and anticholinergics are withheld for 24 hours before the test because they slow the motility of the intestinal tract.

• *During the Test*

The hospitalized patient may return to the nursing unit for an interval before the small bowel filming begins. Obtain instructions from the radiology department about the nothing-by-mouth status or eating a prescribed meal.

• *Posttest*

A laxative is given to help evacuate the barium. Retained barium can cause constipation, obstruction, or fecal impaction.

Inform the patient that the feces will be gray or whitish for 24 to 72 hours until all barium has been evacuated.

The patient should plan to rest for the remainder of the day because the test is tiring.

UREA NITROGEN • SERUM

Synonyms: Blood urea nitrogen, BUN

N O R M A L   V A L U E S

Older adult (>60 years): 8–21 mg/dl *or* SI 2.9–7.5 µmol/L
Child to adult (1–40 years): 5–20 mg/dl *or* SI 1.8–7.1 µmol/L
Infant (birth–1 year): 4–16 mg/dl *or* SI 1.4–5.7 µmol/L

Purpose of the Test

The BUN level is used to evaluate renal function. With serum creatinine, it is used to monitor patients in renal failure or those receiving dialysis therapy. It is part of the routine blood chemistry screen or SMA (sequential multiple analyzer) computer.

The BUN and creatinine are both by-products of protein metabolism and are usually evaluated together. A *BUN/creatinine ratio* expresses the relation. Normally, it is 6–20/1. An increase in the ratio is usually due to overproduction or lower excretion of urea. A decrease is usually due to low protein diets, malnutrition, liver disease, or medications which cause the creatinine level to rise but not the BUN (cimetidine, trimethoprim, tetracycline).

Procedure

A red-topped tube is used to obtain 7 ml of venous blood.

Findings

Increase	*Decrease*
Acute or chronic renal failure	Overhydration
Shock	Starvation
Renal artery stenosis	Intravenous therapy
Hemorrhage	Low-protein diet
Postrenal obstruction	Acromegaly
Stress	Severe liver damage
Congestive heart failure	
Burns	
Increased protein intake	
Dehydration	
Hyperalimentation	
Ketoacidosis	
Long-term steroid therapy	
Diabetes mellitus	

Interfering Factors

None

Nursing Implementation

No specific patient instruction or nursing intervention is needed.

URIC ACID • SERUM

Synonym: Urate

NORMAL VALUES

Adult
  Male: 4.5–8 mg/dl *or* SI 0.27–0.47 µmol/L
  Female: 2.5–6.2 mg/dl *or* SI 0.15–0.37 µmol/L
Child <12 years: 2–5.5 mg/dl *or* SI 0.12–0.32 µmol/L
Adult >60 years
  Male: 4.2–8 mg/dl *or* SI 0.25–0.47 µmol/L
  Female: 2.7–6.8 mg/dl *or* SI 0.16–0.40 µmol/L

Purpose of the Test

Uric acid is the end product of protein metabolism and is excreted from the body by the kidneys and bowel. Uric acid levels are commonly done to assess for hyperuricemia, an elevated level of uric acid in the blood, which results from excessive production of uric acid or impaired excretion of uric acid, or a combination of the two causes. The conditions of abnormal overproduction include the abnormal metabolism of purines and amino acids, excessive catabolism of body tissues, destruction of nucleoproteins, some cancers before and after chemotherapy or radiation, some endocrine and hemolytic disorders, and conditions that cause acidosis or lactic acidosis. Impaired excretion or urate retention is usually due to renal disease that affects tubular secretion and reabsorption. It may also be caused by reduced renal blood flow and decreased renal filtration of the blood.

Gout is a genetic disorder of purine metabolism that usually produces a high level of uric acid in the blood and monosodium urate crystal deposits throughout the body. The deposits are located in the joints, cartilage, bone, bursae, and subcutaneous tissue. The urate crystals can accumulate in the renal pelvis and cause uric acid kidney stones to form. If severe, hyperuricemia can also cause urate crystal accumulation in the renal tubules and ureters, resulting in obstruction and renal failure.

Procedure

A red-topped tube is used to collect 5 to 10 ml of venous blood.

Findings

Increase	*Decrease*
Gout	Falconi's syndrome
Diabetic ketoacidosis	Wilson's disease
Renal failure	Hodgkin's disease
Shock	Multiple myeloma
Polycystic kidney disease	Bronchogenic carcinoma
Down's syndrome	Xanthinuria
Leukemia	
Glycogen storage disease	
Lymphoma	
Lesch-Nyhan's syndrome	
Toxemia of pregnancy	
Hemolytic anemia	

Lead poisoning
Polycythemia vera
Psoriasis
Pernicious anemia
Tumor lysis syndrome

Interfering Factors

Starvation
High purine diet
Stress
Caffeine or vitamin C ingestion

Nursing Implementation

- *Pretest*

When the laboratory protocol specifies a fasting specimen, instruct the patient to discontinue all food and fluid for 8 hours.

On the requisition slip, list all medications taken by the patient. Many drugs cause either a false-positive or false-negative result.

Report ingestion of foods rich in purine (organ meats, legumes, meat, and some fish), strenuous exercise or heavy alcohol ingestion within 24 hours, as this may cause a temporary rise in uric acid levels.

- *Posttest*

No specific nursing intervention is required.

URIC ACID • URINE

Synonyms: None

NORMAL VALUES

Average diet (adult): 250–750 mg/24 hours *or* SI 1.48–4.43 µmol/24 hours
Low purine diet (male): <420 mg/24 hours *or* SI <2.83 µmol/24 hours
Low purine diet (female): <400 mg/24 hours *or* SI <2.36 µmol/24 hours
High purine diet (adult): <1000 mg/24 hours *or* SI <5.9 µmol/24 hours

Purpose of the Test

Urinary uric acid measures the urinary excretion of uric acid in patients with renal calculi or those at risk for the development of a calculus. The test is also used to assess the effect of enzyme deficiency or metabolic abnormality that results in the overproduction of uric acid, especially in certain cancer patients.

When leukemia is treated with cytotoxic drugs or when malignant tumors are irradiated, there is tumor necrosis and a metabolic breakdown of nucleoprotein. The massive amount of uric acid and urate crystal production can cause an acute or dangerous elevation of the urine uric acid level. The urate crystals can block the renal tubules and ureters, resulting in renal failure.

Procedure

A 24-hour urine collection is used to measure the amount of daily uric acid that is excreted.

Findings

Increase	*Decrease*
Uric acid nephrolithiasis	Chronic glomerulonephritis
Viral hepatitis	Collagen disease
Gout	Diabetic glomerulosclerosis
Glycogen storage disease	Lead toxicity
Leukemia (chronic myeloid)	Folic acid deficiency
Lesch-Nyhan's syndrome	Xanthinuria
Acute leukemia of childhood	
Radiation therapy	
Lymphatic leukemia	
Crohn's disease	
Lymphosarcoma	
Ulcerative colitis	
Wilson's disease	
Ileostomy	
Cystinosis	
Surgical jejunoileal bypass	
Sickle cell anemia	
Polycythemia vera	
Tumor lysis syndrome	

Interfering Factors

Failure to collect all urine during the test period
Failure to store the specimen properly
High or low purine diet
Many medications (including aspirin, antiinflammatory drugs,
   diuretics, vitamin C, and x-ray contrast medium)

Nursing Implementation

- *Pretest*

Instruct the patient to collect all urine of the test period and store
it in a large container. Some laboratories require the specimen to
be refrigerated or stored on ice during the test period. Other
laboratories do not require refrigeration, but the specimen container has sodium hydroxide added to maintain alkalinity of the
urine. This prevents precipitation of urate crystals in an acid medium.

- *During the Test*

Have the patient void at 8 a.m. Discard this urine and start the
   test. All urine is collected for 24 hours, including the 8 a.m.
   specimen of the following morning.
Ensure that the label and requisition slip contain the patient's
   name and the time and date of the start and finish of the test.

- *Posttest*

List all medications taken by the patient on the requisition slip.
Arrange for transport of the specimen to the laboratory.

URINALYSIS • URINE

Synonyms: Routine urinalysis, UA

N O R M A L   V A L U E S

Color: yellow, clear
Specific gravity: 1.003–1.029
pH: 4.5–7.8
Protein: negative
Bilirubin: negative
Urobilinogen: normal

(continued)

N O R M A L   V A L U E S   *(continued)*

Glucose: negative
Ketones: negative
Occult blood: negative
RBCs (male): 0–3 per HPF
RBCs (female): 0–5 per HPF
WBCs: 0–5 per HPF
Bacteria: negative
Leukocyte esterase: negative
Casts: 0–4 hyaline casts per LPF
Crystals: few

Purpose of the Test

Urinalysis is performed as part of the routine evaluation of patients on pre-admission or admission to the hospital. Multiple medical problems will produce changes in urine. Urinalysis is an economical and non-invasive method to detect a wide range of disorders. Urinalysis is performed to screen for urinary tract disorders, kidney disorders, urinary neoplasms, and other medical conditions that produce changes in the urine. This test is also used to monitor the effects of treatment of known renal or urinary conditions.

Procedure

A clean container with a lid is used to collect 15 ml or more of urine. A random sample may be used, but the first-voided specimen of the morning is preferred.

Findings

- *Elevated Values*

Specific Gravity

Dehydration
Fever
Profuse sweating
Vomiting, diarrhea, or both
Glycosuria
Proteinuria
Congestive heart failure
Adrenal insufficiency

pH

Metabolic alkalosis
Respiratory alkalosis
Bacteriuria (*Proteus* sp., *Pseudomonas*)
Vegetarian diet
Nasogastric suctioning
Prolonged vomiting
Falconi's syndrome

Altered secretion of antidiuretic hormone

Protein

Nephrotic syndrome
Renal disorders associated with
Hypertension
Diabetes mellitus
Systemic lupus erythematosus
Amyloidosis

Urobilinogen

Hemolytic anemia
Hepatitis (infectious, toxic, chemical)
Cirrhosis
Congestive heart failure

Ketonuria

Acidosis
Alcoholic ketoacidosis
Diabetic ketoacidosis
Fasting or starvation
Increased protein intake

Casts

Glomerulonephritis
Chronic renal disease
Nephrotic syndrome
Bacterial pyelonephritis
Renal failure

Occult Blood

Glomerulonephritis
Urolithiasis
Urinary tract infection
Tumor, benign or malignant
Polycystic kidney
Renal infarct
Lupus nephritis

Milkman's syndrome
Alkali therapy

Bilirubin

Hepatitis (infectious, toxic, chemical)
Biliary obstruction (intrahepatic or extrahepatic)

Glucose

Hyperglycemia
Diabetes mellitus

Crystals

Uric acid crystals
Gout
Rapid nucleic acid turnover
Urolithiasis
Calcium oxalate crystals
Chronic renal failure
Ethylene glycol ingestion
Urolithiasis
Triple phosphate crystals
Obstructive uropathy
Urinary tract infection
Urolithiasis

Red Blood Cells

Benign tumor
Carcinoma
Urinary calculi
Glomerulonephritis
IgA neuropathy
Lupus nephritis
Sclerosis

Occult Blood (cont.)

Goodpasture's syndrome
Benign prostatic hypertrophy
Blood dyscrasia, hemolysis of
   RBCs
Endocarditis
Leukemia
Poison (snake or spider bite)
Parasitic disease
Thermal or crush injury
Trauma
Severe exercise, jogging

Red Blood Cells (cont.)

Urinary tract infection
Trauma from exercise

White Blood Cells

Urinary tract infection (cystitis, prostatitis, urethritis, pyelonephritis)

Bacteria

Chronic urinary tract infection
Pyelonephritis
Cystitis, acute or chronic

- Decreased Values

Specific Gravity

Overhydration
Diuresis
Hypotension
Pyelonephritis
Glomerulonephritis
Renal tubular dysfunction
Severe renal damage
Diabetes insipidus

pH

Metabolic acidosis
Respiratory acidosis
Diabetes mellitus
Diarrhea
Starvation
Emphysema
Renal failure

Interfering Factors

Insufficient quantity of urine (less than 2 ml)
Contamination of the specimen
Prolonged delay before analysis is performed
Warming of the specimen
Metabolites of pyridium
High vitamin C (may cause false low glucose level)
IVP dyes (will affect specific gravity)

Nursing Implementation

- Pretest

Instruct the patient to collect a sample of urine, preferably on rising in the morning. (The specimen must not be contaminated by toilet paper, toilet water, feces, or secretions. Women should not collect urine during menstruation, to prevent contamination with the bloody discharge.)

• *Posttest*

Label the container with the patient's name, the time, and the date of the voiding.

Arrange for transport of the specimen to the laboratory within 30 minutes. If this cannot be accomplished, refrigerate the specimen.

✓ QUALITY CONTROL
Refrigeration preserves the elements of the urine, but the delay can cause crystals to precipitate. If the specimen stands at room temperature, the warmth causes bacteria and WBCs to decompose.

✓ QUALITY CONTROL
Dipsticks used in urinalysis must be kept in closed container at all times. Ambient humidity will decrease the test strip's sensitivity to occult blood and increase its sensitivity to glucose (causing false-positive results).

URINE CULTURE	• URINE

NORMAL VALUES

No growth

Purpose of the Test

Culture of the urine is used to diagnose a urinary tract infection and to monitor the number of microorganisms in the urine.

Procedure

Midstream Catch. A clean-voided midstream technique is used to obtain 15 ml or more of urine in a sterile container. A first voided specimen of the day is used because it has the highest colony count after an overnight incubation period.

Indwelling Catheter. A sterile needle and syringe are used to obtain 4 ml or more of urine from the urine sample port of the catheter. The urine is then placed in a sterile container.

Findings

Positive

Urinary tract infection (*Escherichia coli, Proteus* spp., *Enterobacter* spp., *Pseudomonas, Klebsiella* spp., *Streptococcus faecalis, Staphylococcus aureus, Candida albicans, Mycobacterium* spp.)

Interfering Factors

Contamination of the specimen
Antimicrobial therapy

Nursing Implementation

• *Pretest*

Instruct the patient regarding the proper procedure for collection of a clean-catch midstream urine sample. Before the specimen is collected, hands must be washed with soap and the area surrounding the urinary meatus must be cleansed.

| ✓ QUALITY CONTROL
Contamination of the specimen causes a false-positive result.

• *During the Test*

Midstream or Clean-Catch Method

Female. Instruct the female that after spreading the labia, the perineum, vulva, and urinary meatus are cleansed with three soapy sponges, using one downward stroke for each sponge. Each sponge is used only once and is discarded. Then a sponge with water is used to remove the soap, using the same single downward stroke. After the cleansing is completed, the labia must be maintained in that separated position until after the urine is collected.

Male. Instruct the male to cleanse the urethral meatus with the three soapy sponges and then rinse with the water sponge. Each sponge is used once and discarded. If uncircumcised, the preputial meatus must be retracted and the glans cleansed.

Collecting the Urine

Instruct the patient to begin the urinary stream and void about 1 oz. and then as the urine flow continues, collect the urine by catching it midstream into the container. The first and last parts of the urinary stream are not used for the collection of the specimen. During the collection process, the container must not touch the perineal skin or hair. Once the specimen is obtained, the patient places the lid on the container without touching the inner surfaces.

Indwelling Catheter Method

Clamp the tubing below the urine collection port for 10 minutes. Cleanse the port with an alcohol sponge. Use a sterile needle and syringe to collect the urine sample through this port. Place the urine in a sterile container. Unclamp the tubing.

✓ QUALITY CONTROL

Urine is not collected from the drainage bag because colonized bacteria and bacteria from external sources would contaminate the specimen.

• *Posttest*

Ensure that the requisition slip and the specimen container are properly labeled and sent to the laboratory without delay.

URINE PROTEIN, 24-HOUR • URINE

Synonyms: None

N O R M A L   V A L U E S
40–150 mg/24 hours *or* SI 40–150 mg/24 hours

Purpose of the Test

When proteinuria is detected by urinalysis, it is an indicator of renal disease. As a follow-up study, the 24-hour specimen measures the amount of protein in the urine. Repeat tests may be performed to determine if the problem is intermittent or persistent. Additional tests of renal function will also be done at this time.

Procedure

A 24-hour urine specimen is collected in a large, clear glass or plastic container.

Findings

Glomerulonephritis
Renal transplant rejection
Tubular necrosis
Chronic pyelonephritis
Nephrotic syndrome
Diabetic glomerulosclerosis
Renal failure
Urinary tract infection
Toxemia of pregnancy
Multiple myeloma
Congestive heart failure
Malignant hypertension

Interfering Factors

Contamination of the specimen with mucus, vaginal or prostatic secretions, or white cells
Dilute urine from excessive fluid intake
Failure to collect all urine
Warming of the specimen

Nursing Implementation

- *Pretest*

Instruct the patient to collect all urine for a 24-hour period. The specimen must be refrigerated or kept on ice throughout the test period.
Advise the patient to drink a regular amount of fluids during the test period.

✓ QUALITY CONTROL
Excessive fluid intake will dilute the urine and give a false-negative value.

- *During the Test*

Have the patient void at 8 a.m. and discard the urine.

The test period starts at this time and all urine is collected for 24 hours, including the 8 a.m. specimen of the following morning.

Ensure that the patient's name, and the time and date of the start and finish of the test, are written on the label and requisition slip.

- *Posttest*

Keep the specimen refrigerated until it is transported to the laboratory.

UROBILINOGEN • FECES, URINE

NORMAL VALUES

FECES
Adult: 40–280 mg/day *or* 75–275 Ehrlich Units/100 g

URINE
Adult
Male: 0.3–2.1 mg/2 hours *or* SI 0.5–3.6 µmol/2 hours
Female: 0.1–1.1 mg/2 hours *or* SI 0.2–1.9 µmol/2 hours

Purpose of the Test

Fecal and urinary urobilinogen are used to screen for evidence of hemolytic anemia and to help to confirm the diagnosis of liver disease or biliary tract obstruction.

Procedure

Feces

The procedure may be based upon a single stool specimen, several consecutive daily stool specimens, or a pooled, 4-day specimen.

Urine

The two-hour urine collection is scheduled in the afternoon, between noon and 4 p.m.

Findings

Increase	*Decrease*
Hemolytic anemia (sickle-cell, thalassemia, pernicious)	Massive liver damage (severe cirrhosis, hepatitis)
Hemorrhage into body tissues	Biliary tract obstruction (choledocholithiasis, cancer of the head of the pancreas or common bile duct)
Hemolysis of erythrocytes	
Moderate liver damage	

Interfering Factors

Exposure of specimen to sunlight or warmth
Failure to collect all specimens in the designated time period
Recent or current use of antibiotics

Nursing Implementation

• *Pretest*

Explain the procedure to the patient to maximize cooperation and accuracy in the collection of the specimen.

Feces

All the stool specimen or specimens are to be placed in one or more special, darkened containers, as required by the particular laboratory protocol. The stool specimen must not be contaminated with toilet paper, toilet water, or urine.

Urine

Schedule the test from 2 to 4 p.m. The patient voids just before 2 p.m. and this specimen is discarded.

Give the patient 500 ml of water to drink all at once.

> ✓ QUALITY CONTROL
> When it is exposed to sunlight or the warmth of room temperature, urobilinogen will convert to urobilin. Multiple specimens of feces and all urine specimens are refrigerated in dark containers throughout the test period.

• *During the Test*

Feces

Each total bowel movement is placed in a separate stool container or added into one large container.

Urine

From 2 to 4 p.m., place all voided urine in a dark-colored, sterile urine container.

● *Posttest*

The requisition slip and container(s) for pooled or multiple specimens are labeled with the patient's name, and the dates and times of the specimen collection.

A single, fresh stool specimen is sent to the laboratory immediately.

Continued refrigeration of urine or multiple stool specimens is required when there is a delay in transport of 30 minutes or more.

V

• SERUM

Synonyms: ADH, antidiuretic hormone

NORMAL VALUES

If serum osmolality >290 mOsm/kg: 2–12 pg/ml *or* SI 1.85–11.1 pmol/L
If serum osmolality <290 mOsm/kg: <2 pg/ml *or* SI <1.85 pmol/L

Purpose of the Test

A serum ADH determination is obtained to diagnose diabetes insipidus (DI) and inappropriate secretion of the antidiuretic hormone (SIADH).

Procedure

Venipuncture is performed to obtain 5 ml of blood in a red-topped tube.

Findings

Increase	*Decrease*
SIADH	DI

Interfering Factors

Noncompliance with diet, activity, and medication restrictions
Pain
Stress
Mechanical ventilation
Alcohol
Medications (anesthetics, carbamazepine, chlorothiazide, cyclophosphamide, estrogen, oxytocin, vincristine)

Nursing Implementation

• *Pretest*

Instruct the patient not to eat or drink for 12 hours before the test.

Instruct the patient not to drink alcohol for 24 hours before the test.

Instruct the patient to limit physical activity for 12 hours before the test. The patient should lie down and rest for 30 minutes before the blood is drawn.

Obtain a medication history to determine if any interfering drugs are being taken. Check with the prescriber to determine if these drugs are to be withheld or continued.

Assess the patient for pain and stress, which may interfere with results.

- *During the Test*

Venipuncture is performed.

- *Posttest*

Instruct the patient to resume normal activity and diet. Administer prescribed medications that were withheld for the test.

VENOGRAPHY • RADIOGRAPHY

Synonyms: Phlebography, contrast venography

N O R M A L   V A L U E S

No evidence of intraluminal filling defects, obstruction, incompetent venous valves, calcifications, or dilations of collateral veins

Purpose of the Test

Venography is used to investigate venous function, suspected obstruction, venous insufficiency, postphlebotic syndrome, and the source of pulmonary embolism. It also evaluates veins before and after bypass surgery, reconstructive surgery, or thrombolytic therapy to determine the effectiveness of treatment.

Procedure

Contrast medium is injected into the vein via a butterfly needle or an intravenous catheter. Using a tilt table, fluoroscopy, and x-ray studies, the contrast medium illustrates the flow patterns of the venous circulation and identifies the site of occlusion in the vein.

In venography of the lower extremities, either ascending or descending venography may be used. Ascending venography uses a butterfly needle placed in a small vein on the dorsum of the foot. In descending venography, a catheter is placed in the common femoral vein via a percutaneous femoral approach.

Findings

Deep vein thrombosis
Tumor (extrinsic compression)
Vascular tumor (intrinsic blockage)
Venous compression syndrome
Venous insufficiency
Varicose veins
Congenital malformation
Traumatic injury to the vein

Interfering Factors

Allergy to iodine or contrast medium
Renal failure
Congestive heart failure
Severe pulmonary hypertension

Nursing Implementation

• *Pretest*

Identify any allergy to iodine or shellfish or an allergic reaction to a previous x-ray study that used contrast medium.

Instruct the patient regarding the procedure and pretest preparation. Obtain written consent from the patient or person legally designated to make health care decisions for the patient.

Ensure that the pretest blood urea nitrogen and creatinine determinations are performed and the results are posted in the patient's chart. This is carried out to ensure that renal function is adequate, since the kidneys must clear the contrast material from the body.

Solid foods are omitted for 4 hours before the test, but water is permitted.

Record baseline vital signs.

- *During the Test*

Provide emotional support during the period of discomfort. The injection of contrast material is painful.

Monitor the patient for allergic reaction to the contrast medium.

On completion of the test, an intravenous solution of 200 to 300 ml of heparinized saline is administered. This flushes the contrast medium from the veins.

- *Posttest*

Obtain vital signs and record the results.

Assess the puncture site for signs of swelling, pain, redness, or hematoma. Report any indication of phlebitis.

Keep the patient on bedrest for 2 hours.

Resume the previous dietary status. Instruct the patient to drink extra fluids for 24 hours to help flush the remaining contrast medium from the veins and kidneys. Frequent urination is expected.

VISUAL ACUITY TESTS • VISION TESTS

Synonym: VA

NORMAL VALUES

Distance vision: 20/20 vision or better in each eye
Near vision: 14/14 vision or better in each eye

Purpose of the Test

Visual acuity testing is performed to assess the sharpness of central vision. The test results are written in a fraction form, such as 20/20 vision. The first number or numerator represents the distance between the patient and the Snellen chart (Fig. 7). The second number or denominator represents the lowest line on the Snellen chart that is read correctly by the patient.

Procedure

Distance Vision. Testing each eye separately, the patient is asked to read the lines of the Snellen chart from a distance of 20 ft.

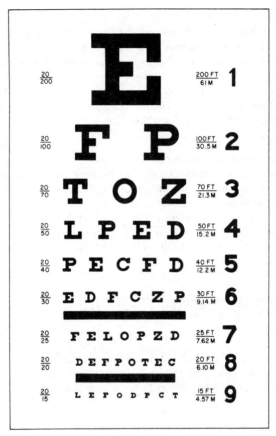

Figure 7. The Snellen Chart.

Near Vision. From a distance of 14 in, the patient is asked to read the small print or identify the location of the opening in each letter c.

Findings

Abnormal Values. Anything other than 20/20 for distance vision or 14/14 for near vision is considered abnormal.

Interfering Factors

Failure to bring corrective lenses to the test
Using improperly prescribed or outdated lenses

Nursing Implementation

• *Pretest*

Place the patient 20 ft from the Snellen chart. The patient may stand or sit for the test. Plan to test the vision without corrective lenses first and then with the corrective lenses used for distance vision.

• *During the Test*

Have the patient occlude the left eye and begin testing the right eye.

Ask the patient to read the letters for each line, starting at the top or starting at a lower line where the patient can see the letters clearly.

If the chart uses the letter E, ask the patient to position the fingers in the same direction as the E on a particular line of the chart. If the chart has numbers or objects, the patient identifies them.

Ask the patient to continue reading the progressively smaller lines until errors are made on more than half the letters or until the line marked 20 is completed.

Repeat the test for the other eye.

If the patient with corrective lenses cannot see the line marked 400 (the large E) from 20 ft away, walk the patient toward the chart until the letter can be identified. Record the distance from the chart. If necessary, assess the ability of the patient to count fingers, see hand movement, or perceive light, usually from a distance of 1 ft.

Near vision: Request that the patient use the corrective lenses to read a sample of tiny print from a distance of 14 in. As an alternative, ask the patient to use a finger to point in the same direction as the opening of the letter C. Each eye is tested separately.

• *Posttest*

Record the results for each eye, without and then with the corrective lenses.

VISUAL FIELD TESTING • VISION TESTS

Synonyms: None

Purpose of the Test

Visual field testing is performed to detect a loss of acuity in part of the central visual field and estimate the location and extent of retinal change. An Amsler grid or a tangent screen may be used.

Amsler Grid. This is a screening test that assesses the central portion of the total visual field (Fig. 8a). When there is deterioration or damage to the central visual field, the fovea centralis, or the macula, the patient may be unable to see the central black dot or may not see all four sides of the grid. Some of the grid may be seen as blurred or distorted instead of the horizontal and vertical black lines that form squares (Fig. 8b).

Tangent Screen Test. This measures the central portion of the visual field by mapping the boundaries of the central vision of each eye. After mapping the perimeter, the optic disc area is located and its boundary is mapped. Since the optic disc has no photoreceptors, it acts like a small blind spot in the central visual field. Once the mapping of the outer and inner boundaries is completed, each eye is tested to verify that there is visual acuity in all areas within the boundaries.

Procedure

The Amsler grid is placed 13 to 14 in from the patient. The vision of each eye is tested separately. The patient is asked to describe what is seen.

The tangent screen hangs on a wall, 40 in from the patient, and the vision of each eye is tested separately. The patient states

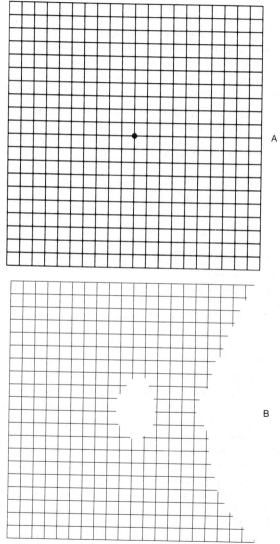

Figure 8. *A,* Amsler grid. *B,* Loss of visibility of some lines or the dot in-dicates retinal abnormality.

when he or she sees the test object, which is a disc with a black side and a white side. Use the black side when the tangent screen has a white background and the white side when the screen has a black background. The results are mapped to define the perimeters of the central visual field and any areas of deficit within the normal field.

Findings

Abnormal Results. These are consistent with macular degeneration, hemianopsia, pituitary tumor, meningioma, cerebral aneurysm, cerebral vascular accident, glaucoma, retinal detachment, and/or retinitis pigmentosa.

Interfering Factors

Severe loss of vision or blindness
Failure to focus on the central dot or object on the map

Nursing Implementation

• *Pretest*

Instruct the patient to wear corrective lenses for each of these tests.
Provide an occluder or a folded tissue to cover one eye as the other eye is tested.

• *During the Test*

Amsler Grid

Place the patient about 13 in from the Amsler grid.
Request that the patient keep his or her eye focused on the black dot.
Ask the patient:
  Is the black dot visible?
  Are the four sides of the grid visible?
  Are all lines and squares visible?
  Repeat the test on the other eye.

Tangent Screen

Ask the patient to sit down for the examination. The chair is placed 40 in from the wall where the screen is hung.
Stand at the side of the screen and observe that the patient's

eye remains centered and does not search for the test object.

Ask the patient to fix his or her eye on the center of the screen and state when the test object first comes into view on the screen.

Use a hand-held wand with the test object on the tip to do the mapping. Along each tangent line, bring the object into view, from the periphery toward the center.

Place a pin on each tangent line where the patient states the test object is first seen. These pins mark the outer boundary of the central visual field.

Identify and map the boundaries of the optic disc. In a small area on the nasal side of each visual field, the patient sees the disc along several tangent lines; first it disappears and then reappears. Mark the places of disappearance and reappearance until the circular area is completed. This is the area of the optic disc.

Now that the boundaries are completed, use the test object to confirm visual acuity throughout the visual field. In each sector defined by the tangent lines, place the black test object on the black field. Turn the test object so that the white side shows. Ask the patient to state when the object appears. Repeat this maneuver in each sector.

If an area is not identified, repeat the maneuver with a test object of a different color or one of a larger size.

Record the results on the special test sheet and then repeat the test on the other eye.

● *Posttest*

No special nursing intervention is required.

VITAMIN D, ACTIVATED ● SERUM OR PLASMA

Synonym: 1,25-dihydroxycholecalciferol

N O R M A L   V A L U E S

25–45 pg/ml *or* SI 60–108 nmol/L

Purpose of the Test

Activated vitamin D levels are assessed to evaluate causes of hypo-calcemia. Vitamin D is derived from the action of ultraviolet light on a group of provitamins in the skin. Vitamin D is also produced from vitamin D-rich food by the liver and kidneys. The vitamin D is first converted in the liver to 25,hydroxycholecalciferol and then to 1,25-dehydroxycholecalciferol in the kidney. Activated vi-tamin D elevates plasma calcium and phosphate levels by increas-ing intestinal absorption of calcium and phosphate and increas-ing the release of calcium from bone into blood.

Procedure

A fasting venous specimen is needed. If a serum level is ordered, 5 ml of blood is collected in a red-topped tube. If a plasma level is desired, 5 ml of blood is collected in a green-topped tube.

Findings

Increase	*Decrease*
Hyperparathyroidism	Anticonvulsants
Overdose of vitamin D	Hepatic failure
Sarcoidosis	Hypoparathyroidism
	Isoniazid
	Malabsorption syndrome
	Osteomalacia
	Pseudohypoparathyroidism
	Renal failure

Interfering Factors

Phosphorus deficiency
Prolonged lack of exposure to sunlight

Nursing Implementation

The nurse performs actions similar to those in other venipunc-ture procedures.

• *Pretest*

Instruct the patient not to eat or drink for 8 hours before the test.

WATER DEPRIVATION TEST • URINE

Synonyms: Dehydration test, concentration test

NORMAL VALUES

Specific gravity: 1.025–1.032
Osmolality: >800 mOsm/kg *or* SI >800 mmol/kg

Purpose of the Test

Normally, as fluid intake is withheld, blood osmolality increases and urine output decreases, whereas urinary osmolality increases. The increase in serum osmolality causes an increase in ADH secretion. The water deprivation test is performed to diagnose diabetes insipidus (DI) and to assess the kidney's ability to concentrate urine based on extracellular fluid load. In patients with DI, there is not a normal response to increased plasma osmolality; instead, little or no increase in ADH occurs, resulting in little or no change in urinary output or osmolality.

As part of the water deprivation test, a *vasopressin stimulation test* or *vasopressin test* may be performed to distinguish between neurogenic and nephrogenic DI. This distinction is important in determining appropriate treatment plans.

Procedure

During the test, the patient is deprived of fluid intake and periodic urine specimens are obtained for osmolality and specific gravity determinations. The urine is collected in separate clean containers and placed on ice or refrigerated. Strict urinary output measurements are maintained.

If a vasopressin stimulation test is included, hypertonic saline or nicotine is given to stimulate ADH release. If complete neurogenic DI is present, no change is noted on urinary output or osmolality. If partial neurogenic DI is present, only minor changes occur. If desired, a vasopressin test may be performed. After vasopressin is given, no change will occur in urinary output or osmolality if nephrogenic DI is present. With central DI, the urine osmolality will increase and urinary output will decrease.

Findings

If there is no change in urine osmolality, the diagnosis is DI.

Interfering Factors

Noncompliance with fluid restrictions
Inability to complete test because of hypovolemia
Glucosuria
Administration of radiopaque dyes within 7 days

Nursing Implementation

• *Pretest*

Assess patient's hemodynamic status. If vasopressin test is planned, check for a history of coronary artery disease, as vasopressin may cause coronary artery spasm.

Obtain baseline serum and urine specimens for osmolality determinations.

Baseline weight is obtained before the evening meal on the day before testing.

• *During the Test*

Assess the patient for hypovolemia (tachycardia, orthostatic hypotension).

Observe the patient to ensure compliance with the nothing-by-mouth status.

Obtain a urine specimen every 2 hours. Label each specimen with the time and the amount obtained. Document urinary output.

Weigh patient every 2 to 4 hours. Maintain the patient on the nothing-by-mouth status until 2 to 5% of the patient's weight is lost (takes approximately 6 to 12 hours).

After 2 to 5% of body weight is lost and urinary output continues with urinary osmolality plateauing, an ADH stimulation test may be performed by administering hypertonic saline (3% sodium chloride) or nicotine as ordered.

Continue to collect urine specimens for amount and osmolality.

If a vasopressin test is to be performed, check the patient's blood pressure and document; notify the physician if the patient is hypertensive. Aqueous vasopressin is given subcutaneously or intravenously. Collect the urine specimen for the amount and osmolality 1 hour after vasopressin administration. Another method is to give long-acting vasopressin in oil intramuscularly the night before the test. Urine is collected in the morning three times at hourly intervals. This method cannot be performed in conjunction with the water deprivation test.

⊘ **COMPLICATION ALERT** ⊘ Hypovolemia may occur with the water deprivation test. Patients with DI will continue to put urine out even though they have no fluid intake. Observe the patient carefully for hypovolemia (tachycardia and hypotension). If a vasopressin test is performed, the administration of vasopressin may produce the complications of high blood pressure or coronary artery spasms, or both. Monitor the patient's blood pressure, listen for complaints of chest pain or discomfort. If on a monitor, check for ST changes.

WATER-LOADING TEST	• PLASMA AND URINE

Synonyms: None

N O R M A L   V A L U E S

Urinary output increases and plasma and urine osmolality decrease.

Purpose of the Test

Normally, with an increase in fluid intake, urinary output will increase to maintain a normal plasma osmolality. As the urine volume increases, its osmolality decreases. However, patients with inappropriate secretion of the antidiuretic hormone (SIADH) will not respond to increasing fluid intake. The water-loading test is done if SIADH is suspected.

Procedure

With the water-loading test, the patient orally ingests a water load of 20 to 25 ml/kg body weight. Hourly serum and urine osmolality and urine outputs are recorded for 4 hours.

Findings

Little or no change in urinary output or plasma and urine osmolality readings supports the diagnosis of SIADH.

Interfering Factors

Patient is unable to drink required volume of fluid
Medications (demeclocycline, diuretics, lithium)

Nursing Implementation

- *Pretest*

Assess the patient for hyponatremia.
Obtain a cardiac history on the patient, the results of which may require that the test be cancelled.
Weigh the patient.

- *During the Test*

Instruct the patient to drink the required fluid.
Obtain hourly output measurements and send blood and urine to the laboratory for osmolality determination. On the requisition slip, indicate the hour of the specimen, with zero hour being the time the patient ingested the fluid. See discussion of plasma and urine osmolality for the nursing procedures associated with the collection of these samples.
Observe the patient for water intoxication.

- *Posttest*

Weigh the patient.

✪ **COMPLICATION ALERT** ✪ When patients with SIADH undergo the water-loading test, their output is not increased. The increased fluid load in the extracellular fluid can cause a dilutional hyponatremia. Assess the patient for lethargy, confusion, stupor, muscular twitching, convulsions, and coma.

WHITE BLOOD CELL DIFFERENTIAL   • BLOOD

N O R M A L   V A L U E S

Segmented Neutrophils
Mean percent: 56% *or* SI 0.56 (mean number fraction)
Cell count (range): 1800–7800/μl *or* SI 1.8–7.8 × 10⁹/L

Bands
Mean percent: 3% *or* SI 0.03 (mean number fraction)
Cell count (range): 0–700/μl *or* SI 0–0.07 × 10⁹/L

Eosinophils
Mean percent: 2.7% *or* SI 0.027 (mean number fraction)
Cell count (range): 0–450/μl *or* SI 0–0.45 × 10⁹/L

Basophils
Mean percent: 0.3% *or* SI 0.003 (mean number fraction)
Cell count (range): 0–200/μl *or* SI 0–0.2 × 10⁹/L

Lymphocytes
Mean percent: 34% *or* SI 0.34 (mean number fraction)
Cell count (range): 1000–4800/μl *or* SI 1–4.8 × 10⁹/L

Monocytes
Mean percent: 4% *or* SI 0.04 (mean number fraction)
Cell count (range): 0–800/μl *or* SI 0–0.8 × 10⁹/L

Purpose of the Test

The WBC differential assesses the ability of the body to respond to and eliminate infection. It also detects the severity of infection, allergic reactions, and parasitic infection and identifies various stages of leukemia.

Procedure

A purple-topped tube with EDTA is used to collect 7 ml of venous blood. As an alternative, two purple-tipped capillary tubes can be used to collect blood from a heelstick, earlobe, or finger puncture.

For the peripheral blood smear, two slides with coverslips are prepared immediately using drops of venous or capillary blood.

✓ QUALITY CONTROL

With venipuncture, the tourniquet should be tied lightly for a brief time to prevent pooling of cells in the vein at the site of blood collection. To avoid hemolysis, venipuncture technique must be smooth, with a blood flow that fills the vacuum tube readily. After the blood is collected, the tube is inverted gently 5 to 10 times to mix the anticoagulant and prevent clotting.

Findings

Increase

Neutrophils. Leukemia, bacterial infection, rheumatic fever, severe burns, ketoacidosis, cancer, Downs syndrome

Eosinophils. Pemphigus, eczema, trichinosis, scarlet fever, leukemia, Hodgkin's disease, cancer, rheumatoid arthritis, arcoidosis, allergy, *Echinococcus* disease

Basophils. Hypersensitivity reaction, ulcerative colitis, chronic hemolytic anemia, Hodgkin's disease, myxedema, leukemia, polycythemia vera

Lymphocytes. Infectious mononucleosis, hepatitis, cytomegalovirus infection, pertussis, tuberculosis, syphilis, leukemia

Monocytes. Acute infection, tuberculosis, sarcoidosis, ulcerative colitis, leukemia, multiple myeloma, Hodgkin's disease, non-Hodgkin lymphoma, rheumatoid arthritis

Decrease

Neutrophils. Infection, drug reaction, maternal antibody production, aplastic anemia, leukemia

Eosinophils. Allergies, infection, shock, postoperative response

Basophils. Hyperthyroidism, pregnancy, stress, Cushing's syndrome

Lymphocytes. Heart failure, Hodgkin's disease, systemic lupus erythematosus, aplastic anemia, HIV infection, renal failure, cancer

Monocytes. Bone marrow failure, aplastic anemia

Interfering Factors

Temperature changes
Exercise
Pregnancy
Pain
Mental or physical stress
Heightened emotion

Nursing Implementation

• *Pretest*

Instruct the physically active patient to avoid strenuous activity for 24 hours before the test. Calm the crying infant and relieve pain or distress experienced by the patient.

• *Posttest*

Arrange for prompt transport of the blood to the laboratory.

✓ QUALITY CONTROL
If the blood remains standing in the tube, deterioration of the cells begins within 30 minutes. The nuclei and cytoplasm of the leukocytes are affected.

WOUND CULTURE • SECRETIONS

N O R M A L   V A L U E S
No growth

Purpose of the Test

The wound culture is used to determine the presence of infection and to identify the causative organism.

Procedure

A syringe and needle can be used to aspirate purulent material from a wound. Sterile swabs may also be used to absorb purulent matter from within a draining wound or fistula. For transport to the laboratory, the swabs are placed in a tube that contains culture medium.

Findings

Positive

Staphylococcus aureus
Pseudomonas spp.
Streptococcus pyogenes
Bacteroides spp.
Staphylococcus epidermidis
Clostridium spp.
Escherichia coli
Group D streptococci
Proteus spp.
Klebsiella spp.

Interfering Factors

Antibiotic therapy
Contamination of the specimen

Nursing Implementation

- *Pretest*

If possible, schedule this procedure before antibiotic therapy is started.

Explain that there is only minor discomfort as an open wound is swabbed. If an abscessed area must be opened surgically or a tissue biopsy, debridement, or tissue scraping is required, a local anesthetic may be used. A written consent is needed for these surgical procedures.

- *During the Test*

To express the purulent material, the tissue surrounding the wound is pressed. The cotton swab absorbs the fluid that appears.

The swab may also be inserted into the open lesion or drainage tract. Once the swab is in place, it is rotated against the side walls of the tissue.

A needle and syringe may be used to aspirate fluid from the purulent area or the drainage tract.

✓ QUALITY CONTROL
Ensure that the needle or swab does not touch the skin near the site of infection. The contamination of the specimen with surface organisms produces invalid results.

- *Posttest*

Ensure that the requisition slip indicates the patient's name and age, specific culture site, time, date, clinical diagnosis, and any current antibiotic therapy.

Arrange for prompt transport of the specimen to the laboratory.

✓ QUALITY CONTROL
A delay in starting the culture growth can produce a reduced yield of microorganisms.

X

NORMAL VALUES

Within normal limits. No abnormalities are noted.

Purpose of the Test

The x-ray images identify changes in the postion, size, contour, structure, and density of organs and tissues. X-ray may be used for diagnosis, screening, or evaluation of healing.

Procedure

In the imaging process, the x-ray beam passes through the patient onto the x-ray film. Front, back, side, or oblique views are obtained by changing the patient's position.

Findings

Chest and Heart

Pneumothorax
Pneumonia
Atelectasis
Tuberculosis
Pleural effusion
Pulmonary abscess
Fracture
Scoliosis
Cystic or pulmonary fibrosis
Chronic obstructive pulmonary disease
Tumor
Cyst
Mediastinal nodes
Atherosclerosis

Aortic aneurysm
Congestive heart failure
Cardiac hypertrophy

Intestinal Tract

Perforation
Subphrenic abscess
Obstruction
Foreign body
Ileus
Volvulus
Intussusception
Biliary tract calculus

Urinary System

Renal abscess
Congenital malformation
Renal tuberculosis
Tumor
Cyst
Pyelonephritis
Renal or ureteral calculus
Glomerulonephritis
Polycystic kidney
Hydronephrosis
Hematoma
Amyloidosis

Bones and Joints

Fracture
Dislocation
Subluxation
Gout
Arthritis
Bone cyst or tumor
Osteomyelitis
Osteoporosis
Rickets
Osteomalacia
Paget's disease

Skull

Congenital anomaly
Fracture
Paget's disease
Acromegaly
Osteomyelitis

Spinal Vertebrae

Ankylosing spondylitis
Fracture
Scoliosis
Kyphosis
Ruptured disc
Osteoarthritis
Osteoporosis
Tuberculosis
Paget's disease

Interfering Factors

Excessive movement
Failure to remove metal or jewelry
For abdominal and kidney-ureter-bladder films: retained barium or contrast medium, feces, ascites, gas, obesity

Nursing Implementation

• *Pretest*

Schedule the abdominal or kidney-ureter-bladder film before any radiologic study that uses barium or contrast medium.
For most imaging procedures, instruct the patient to remove all clothes and put on a hospital gown.
Instruct the patient to remove all jewelry and metallic objects from the area that is to be imaged.
Provide reassurance to the patient.

• *During the Test*

Ensure the patient's safety at all times, particularly regarding a potential fall.
Position the patient for the specific views needed.
Instruct the patient to remain motionless during the imaging.

Sometimes the patient is instructed to inhale deeply and hold the breath until the image is taken.

- *Posttest*

Assist the patient in dismounting from the radiography table and getting dressed, as needed.

Bibliography

Adler, A.M., & Carlton, R.R. (1994). *Introduction to radiography and patient care.* Phila: W.B. Saunders.

Alving, B.M., & Griffin, J.H. (1995). Venous thrombosis: How to make the best use of the laboratory to guide therapy. *Consultant, 35*(1), 64–66, 69–71.

Atkin, W.S., Cuzick, J., Northover, J.M.A., et al. (1993). Prevention of colorectal cancer by once-only sigmoidoscopy. *Lancet, 341,* 736–740.

Baer, D.M. (1995). Tips from clinical experts: Assays on bile specimens. *Medical Laboratory Observer, 27*(10), 17–18.

Baer, D.M. (1995). Tips from clinical experts: Fecal fat. *Medical Laboratory Observer, 26*(11), 18, 20.

Baer, D.M. (1995). Tips on technology: Elevated lipase. *Medical Laboratory Observer, 27*(7), 9, 12.

Barrios, F., & Jain, L. (1996). Current concepts in neonatal hyperbilirubinemia. *Neonatal Intensive Care, 9*(3), 48–52.

Bentz, J.S. (1995). Neurology I. Laboratory investigation of multiple sclerosis. *Laboratory Medicine, 26*(6), 293–299.

Bick, R. (1994). Oral anticoagulants and the INR: Confusion, controversy, fiction and fact. *American Clinical Laboratory, 13,* 36–38.

Bick, R.L. (1995). Oral anticoagulants in thrombophlebotic disease. *Laboratory Medicine, 26*(3), 188–193.

Brown, D.R., Kulter, D., Rai, B., et al. (1993). Bacterial concentration and blood volume required for positive blood culture. *Journal of Perinatology, 15,* 157–159.

Brown, K.A. (1996). Hematology II. Glucose-6-phosphate dehydrogenase deficiency and other enzyme defects. *Laboratory Medicine, 27*(6), 390–395.

Brunzel, N.A. (1994). *Fundamentals of urine and body fluid analysis.* Phila: W.B. Saunders.

Bussey, H.I., Force, R.W., Bianco, T.M., et al. (1992). Reliance on prothrombin time ratios causes significant errors in anticoagulation therapy. *Archives of Internal Medicine, 152,* 278–282.

Buyske, J., MacKarem, G., Ulmer, B.C., et al. (1996). Breast cancer in the nineties. *AORN Journal, 64*(1), 64–65, 67–72.

Carter, S., Carter, J.B., & James, K. (1995). Rapid HIV-1 antibody screening. *Laboratory Medicine, 26*(5), 339–342.

Cassetta, R.A. (1993). Sickle cell guidelines stress screening. *American Nurse, 25*(6), 9.

Chernecky, C.C., & Berger, B.J. (Eds.). (1997). *Laboratory tests and diagnostic procedures.* Phila: W.B. Saunders.

Chintapalli, K.N., & Schnitker, J.B. (1994). Spleen imaging. *Applied Radiology, 23*(12), 29–37.

Cohen, S.M., Wexner, S.D., Binderow, S.R., et al. (1994). A prospective randomized endoscopic-blinded trial comparing precolonoscopy bowel cleansing methods. *Diseases of the Colon and Rectum, 37*(7), 689–696.

Coles, M., & Caldwell, S.H. (1995). Diagnostic laporoscopy of the liver and peritoneum using conscious sedation. *Gastroenterology Nursing, 18*(2), 62–66.

Covington, C., Grelegham, P., Board, F., et al. (1996). Family care related to alpha-fetoprotein screening. *Journal of Obstetric, Gynecologic, and Neonatal Nursing, 25*(2), 125–130.

Cozad, J. (1996). Infectious mononucleosis. *Nurse Practitioner: American Journal of Primary Care, 21*(3), 14, 16, 23.

Denison, A.V., & Shum, S.Y. (1995). The evolution of targeted populations in school-based tuberculin testing program. *Image: Journal of Nursing Scholarship, 27*(4), 263–266.

Fleischer, A.C., & Kepple, D.M. (1995). *Diagnostic sonography: Principles and clinical applications* (2nd ed.). Phila: W.B. Saunders.

Fleming, N. (1996). Chemistry: Automated microalbumin assay using Abbott Spectrum. *Laboratory Medicine, 27*(5), 339–341.

Fye, K.H. (1993). Rheumatic diseases: Making the best use of the lab: What results do—and don't—tell you. *Consultant, 33*(4), 133–136, 139–140.

Goodman, L.R., & Putman, C.E. (1992). *Critical care imaging* (3rd ed.). Phila: W.B. Saunders.

Hartwig, P.A. (1993). Patient education for endoscopy. *Seminars for Perioperative Nursing, 2*(3), 187–192.

Havlik, D., & Woods, G.L. (1995). Screening sputum specimens for mycobacterial culture. *Laboratory Medicine, 26*(6), 411–413.

Hayes, D.F. (1993). Tumor markers for breast cancer. *Annals of Oncology, 4,* 807–819.

Hebdon, B., & Letourneau, J.G. (1994). Duplex sonography of extremity arteries and veins. Part 2. *Applied Radiology, 23*(4), 39–48.

Henry, J.B. (1996). *Clinical diagnosis and management by laboratory methods* (19th ed.). Phila: W.B. Saunders.

Herlong, H.F. (1994). Approach to the patient with abnormal liver enzymes. *Hospital Practice, 29*(11), 32–38.

Jackson, M., & Rymer, T.E. (1994). Commentary on viral hepatitis: Anatomy of a diagnosis. *American Journal of Nursing, 94*(1), 43–48.

Jacobs, D.S., Demott, W.R., & Grady, H.J., et al. (Eds.). (1996). *Laboratory test handbook* (4th ed.). Hudson: Lexi-Comp.

Jeffs, M., Cracchiolo-Caraway, A., Lampman, L., et al. (1995). Emotional distress reported by women and husbands prior to a breast biopsy. *Nursing Research, 44*(4), 196–201.

Kelly, P., & Windslow, E.H. (1996). Needle wire localization for nonpalpable breast lesions: Sensations, anxiety levels and informational needs. *Oncology Nursing Forum, 23*(4), 639–645.

Koepke, J.A. (1994). D-dimer test. *Medical Laboratory Observer, 26*(9), 12.

Koepke, J.A. (1995). Tips from the clinical experts: Estimating platelets on peripheral blood. *Medical Laboratory Observer, 27*(11), 20.

Kottke, T.E., Trapp, M.A., Forbes, M.M., et al. (1995). Cancer screening behaviors and attitudes of women in southeastern Minnesota. *Journal of the American Medical Association, 273*(14), 1099–1105.

Krenzischek, D.A., & Tanesco, F.V. (1996). Comparative study of bedside and laboratory measurements of hemoglobin. *American Journal of Critical Care, 5,* 427–432.

Levine, M.S. (1994). The upper GI series: A call to arms. *Applied Radiology, 23*(4), 8.

Lum, G. (1995). Low activities of aspartate and alanine aminotransferase: Their significance in alcoholic liver disease. *Laboratory Medicine, 26*(4), 273–276.

Mahon, S.M. (1995). Prevention and early detection of cancer in women. *Seminars in Oncology Nursing, 11*(2), 88–102.

Mandel, J.S., Bond, J., Church, T.R., et al. (1993). Reducing mortality from colorectal cancer by screening for fecal occult blood. *New England Journal of Medicine, 328,* 1365–1371.

Marchiondo, K. (1994). Pharmacologic stress testing: An alternative to exercise. *Critical Care Nurse, 14*(6), 41–45.

McLeary, R.D. (1995). Transrectal ultrasound of the prostate. *Applied Radiology, 24*(3), 13–18.

Mettler, F.A. (1996). *Esentials of radiology.* Phila: W.B. Saunders.

Michael, P.L., & Glickman, R.A. (1994). Fever of unknown origin: How the causes and workup differ in the elderly. *Consultant, 34*(12), 1665–1666, 1671–1672, 1677–1680.

Morse, E.E., Panek, S., Pisciotto, P., et al. (1993). Reemergence of the international normalized ratio for the standardization of prothrombin time. *Annals of Clinical Laboratory Science, 23,* 184–188.

Muscarella, L.F. (1996). High-level disinfection or "sterilization" of endoscopes? *Infection Control and Hospital Epidemiology, 17*(3), 183–187.

Norris, M.K.G. (1993). Measuring serum amylase levels. *Nursing, 23*(11), 28.

Northouse, L.L., Jeffs, M., Cracchiolo-Caraway, A., et al. (1995). Emotional distress reported by women and husbands prior to a breast biopsy. *Nursing Research, 44*(4), 196–201.

Novak, R., Sandowski, L., Klespies, S.L., et al. (1995). How useful are fecal neutrophil determinations? *Laboratory Medicine, 26*(11), 743–745.

Oesterling, J.E., Jacobsen, S.J., Chute, C.G., et al. (1993). Serum prostate antigen in a community based population of healthy men. *Journal of the American Medical Association, 270,* 860–864.

Otto, C.M., & Pearlman, A.S. (1995). *Textbook of clinical echocardiography.* Phila: W.B. Saunders.

Paisley, J.W., & Lauer, B.A. (1994). Pediatric blood cultures. *Clinics in Laboratory Medicine, 14,* 17–30.

Peake, G., & Muncer, P. (1996). Gynaecological tests. *Practice Nurse, 11*(4), 251–254.

Pepe, J.L. (1993). Diagnostic techniques in blunt and penetrating trauma. *Topics in Emergency Medicine, 15*(1), 8–21.

Peterson, K.L., & Nicod, P. (1997). *Cardiac catherization methods, diagnosis, and therapy.* Phila: W.B. Saunders.

Pfeifer, D.G. (1995). The role of sonography in diagnosing and treating female infertility. *Journal of Diagnostic Medical Sonography, 11*(2), 61–66.

Post-White, J. (1996). The immune system. *Seminars in Oncology Nursing, 12*(2), 89–96.

Ravel, R. (1995). *Clinical laboratory medicine: Clinical application of laboratory data* (6th ed.). St. Louis: Mosby.

Rose, N.C., & Mennuti, M. (1993). Maternal serum screening for neural tube defects and fetal chromasome abnormalities. *Western Journal of Medicine, 159*(3), 312–317.

Saxena, S., Kurola, J., Fong, T., et al. (1995). Are gender specific ALT cutoff values necessary? *Laboratory Medicine, 26*(10), 682–686.

Schapira, D.V., & Levine, R.B., (1996). Breast cancer screening and compliance and evaluation of lesions. *Medical Clinics of North America, 80*(1), 15–26.

Schlager, T.A., Smith, D.E., and Donowitz, L.G. (1995). Are clean-catch urine specimens contaminated less often than nonclean-catch specimens? *Pediatric Infectious Diseases Journal, 14*(10), 909–911.

Schutze, G.E., Rice, T.D., & Starke, J.R. (1993). Routine tuberculin screening of children during hospitalization. *Pediatric Infectious Diseases Journal, 12*(1), 29–32.

Selby, J.V. (1993). Disease prevention: Screening sigmoidoscopy for colorectal cancer. *Lancet, 341,* 728–729.

Selig, P.M. (1996). Pearls for practice: Management of anticoagulation therapy with the international normalized ratio. *Journal of the American Academy of Nurse Practitioners, 8*(2), 77–80.

Siconolfi, L.A. (1995). Clarifying the complexity of liver function tests. *Nursing, 25*(5), 39–44.

Slater, C.A., Davis, R.B., & Shmerling, R.H. (1996). Antinuclear antibody testing: A study of clinical utility. *Archives of Internal Medicine, 156,* 1421–1425.

Slowey, K.B., Slowey, M.J., & Cato, J. (1996). Cardiac complications of laparoscopy: Anesthetic implications. *CRNA: The Clinical Forum for Nurse Anesthetists, 7*(1), 9–13.

Snopek, A.M. (1992). *Fundamentals of special radiographic procedures* (3rd ed.). Phila: W.B. Saunders.

Spiegal, T. (1995). Flexible sigmoidoscopy training for nurses. *Gastroenterology Nursing, 18*(6), 206–209.

Statland, B.E. (1993). Urine albumin. *Medical Laboratory Observer, 25*(1), 14.

Statland, B.E. (1995). Tips from the clinical experts: High alkaline phosphatase. *Medical Laboratory Observer, 27*(10), 17.

Strimike, C. (1996). Understanding intravascular ultrasound. *American Journal of Nursing, 96*(6), 40–43.

Stubbs, J.R. (1996). Coagulation for blood bankers. *Clinics in Laboratory Medicine, 16*(4), 837–871.

Tamaino-Brunner, C., Freda, M.C., & Runowicz, C.D. (1996). "I hope I don't have cancer": Colposcopy and minority women. *Oncology Nursing Forum, 23*(1), 39–44.

Thomas, D.L., & Quinn, T.C. (1993). Serologic testing for sexually transmitted diseases. *Infectious Disease Clinics of North America, 7*(4), 793–824.

Tietz, N.W. (1995). *Clinical guide to laboratory tests* (3rd ed.). Phila: W.B. Saunders.

Torres, L.S. (1993). *Basic medical techniques and patient care for radiologic technologists* (4th ed.). Phila: J.B. Lippincott.

Wagner, H.N., Szabo, Z., & Buchanan, J.W. (1995). *Principles of nuclear medicine.* Phila: W.B. Saunders.

Waldman, A.R., & Osborne, D.M. (1994). Screening for prostate cancer. *Oncology Nursing Forum, 21*(9), 1512–1517.

Williamson, M.R. (1996). *Essentials of ultrasound.* Phila: W.B. Saunders.

Winawer, S.J. (1993). Colorectal cancer screening comes of age. *New England Journal of Medicine, 328,* 416–417.

Winchester, C.B., Dhekne, R.D., Moore, W.H., et al. (1994). Clinical applications of nuclear medicine in gastroenterology. *Gastroenterology Nursing, 17*(1), 20–26.

Woeber, K.A. (1995). Cost-effective evaluation of the patient with a thyroid nodule. *Surgical Clinics of North America, 75*(3), 357.

Wolfson, A.B., & Paris, P.M. (1996). *Diagnostic testing in emergency medicine.* Phila: W.B. Saunders.

Woods, G.L. (1994). TB testing: Methods and time targets . . . Tuberculosis (TB). *Medical Laboratory Observer, 26*(3), 25–28.

Woods, G.L. (1995). Update on laboratory diagnosis of sexually transmitted diseases. *Clinics in Laboratory Medicine, 15*(3), 665–684.

Wright, C.J., & Mueller, C.B. (1995). Screening mammography and public health policy: The need for perspective. *Lancet, 346,* 29–32.

Wright, L. (1994). Prenatal diagnosis in the 1990's. *Journal of Obstetric, Gynecologic, and Neonatal Nursing, 23*(6), 506–515.

Zaloga, G.P. (1993). Reagent testing: Rapid, accurate, urine testing at the bedside . . . Part 1. *Consultant, 33*(6), 90–92, 95–98.

Index

365